Sirt Food Diet

DEBRA SUDWORTH

Table Of Contents

Introduction

Each new year brings with it a new slimming program, and this year many of the eye-grabbing headlines have been of one that allows you to consume healthily and tastefully - occasionally indulge in candy and red wine - without measuring calories, whilst reducing weight and holding away much of the ravages of age. Those findings were a little simplistic, and so were discarded by some, but in fact that was on the back of amazing findings being carried out by nutritional scientists Aidan Goggins and Glenn Matten into what is now called Sirt foods, which have now brought out The Sirt Food Diet.

Scientists discovered back in 2003 that some foods contain compounds with the ability to switch on 'skinny genes' called Sirtuins that are otherwise only activated when we are fasting and exercising. They are not only responsible for burning fat and controlling appetite, but also for cell defense and repair, and as such encourage muscle building - most weight loss regimes result in muscle loss - and heart safety, thus helping to prevent degenerative and inflammatory disorders such as osteoporosis, arthritis, diabetes and probably some cancers.

We all realize that fried meat should be avoided and that red meat should be kept once or twice a week, but poultry, eggs (and milk in moderation) are good, as are lentils, corn, beans, and nuts, of course. Sirt foods do have an especially beneficial omega three oils relationship, which includes oily fish two or three times a week.

CHAPTER 1: THE FUNDAMENTALS OF SIRT FOOD DIET

1.1 What are the Sirt foods?

Trendy new diets appear to pop up regularly, and one of the latest is the Sirt food Diet. This has been a favorite of Europe's actors and is renowned for its red wine and chocolate inclusions. Its founders claim that it's not a fad, but that "Sirt foods" are the secret to unlocking fat loss and disease prevention.

Sirt food Diet:

Sirt food Diet was developed by two celebrity nutritionists working for a private gym in the UK.

They market the diet as a groundbreaking modern lifestyle and wellness program that works by flipping the "skinny gene" on.

This diet is focused on Sirtuin research (SIRTs), a community of seven proteins contained in the body that has been shown to control a number of functions, including metabolism, inflammation, and lifespan;

Some natural plant compounds can increase the amount of these proteins in the body, and the foods they contain have been dubbed "Sirt foods."

The diet incorporates Sirt foods and calorie restriction, which can all cause the body to generate higher Sirtuin rates.

The book of Sirt food Diet contains meal plans and recipes to obey, but there are loads of other books on Sirt food Diet Recipes.

Is It Effective?

The creators of the diet claim that following the Sirt food diet will result in maintaining muscle mass while weight loss and protect you from chronic illness.

Once you've completed the diet, you're encouraged to continue your regular diet, including Sirt foods and the signature green juice of the diet.

The Sirt food Diet's writers make ambitious promises, claiming that the diet will induce super-charge weight loss, turn the "skinny gene" on and avoid disease.

The thing is they don't have any evidence to back them up.

There is no compelling proof to date that the Sirt food Diet has a more positive impact on weight loss than any other diet-restricted by calories.

And while many of those products have medicinal properties, no long-term clinical trials have been performed to establish if consuming a diet abundant in Sirt products has any measurable health benefits.

Nevertheless, a pilot study carried out by the writers and involving 39 participants from their fitness center is published in the Sirt food Diet journal. Nevertheless, the findings of this analysis do not seem to have been published elsewhere.

Goggins, A. and Matten, G., 2005. The Sirt Food Diet.

Participants followed the diet for a week and were exercising daily. Participants weighed a total of 7 pounds (3.2 kg) at the end of the week and retained or even added muscle mass.

These tests, though, are hardly unexpected. Limiting your calorie consumption to 1,000 calories, and concurrently exercising would almost certainly induce weight loss.

Regardless, this kind of rapid weight loss is neither genuine nor long-lasting, and after the first week, this study did not follow participants to see if they gained any of the weight back, which is typically so.

As well as consuming fat and tissue, when the body is drained of nutrition, it utilizes its emergency energy reserves of glycogen.

Each glycogen molecule requires 3–4 water molecules for storage. When your body uses glycogen, that water also gets rid of it. It is known as "weight in water."

Weight loss from fat is one third during the first week of extreme calorie restriction, while the rest come from water, muscle, and glycogen.

Your body must replenish its glycogen reserves as long as the calorie consumption rises, and the weight comes straight back.

Unfortunately, this form of calorie restriction will often cause the body to reduce its metabolic rate, allowing energy levels to be much smaller in calories a day.

This plan is going to help you shed a few pounds at the beginning, but it'll possibly return as soon as the plan is done.

On the other hand, it may very well be a good idea to add Sirt food to your regular diet over the long term. But you may as well miss the diet in that situation, and start practicing it now.

Are Sirt foods Healthy and Sustainable?

Sirt foods are almost always safe options, and thanks to their antioxidant or anti-inflammatory effects, they may also provide certain health benefits.

Yet eating only a handful of particularly healthy foods can not satisfy all the nutritional needs of your body.

Additionally, consuming just 1,000 calories is not usually advised without a doctor's supervision. To certain individuals, only consuming 1,500 calories a day seems too limiting.

In fact, the diet includes up to three green juices a day. While juices can be a good source of vitamins and minerals, they are also a source of sugar and provide almost none of the nutritious fibers that entire fruits and vegetables do.

What's more, all-day sipping on juice is a terrible thing for both your blood sugar and your teeth.

Not to mention, since the diet is so limited in calories and food choices, protein, vitamins, and minerals are more than likely deficient, especially during the first phase.

One positive thing about the diet is that all the foods you can eat on the plan are good for you, which means your overall intake of vitamins, minerals, and nutrients will probably be high.

Some diet that leaves out entire food classes, however, may be risky. Scientists says that 'It's not very really good evidence that confirms the notion of flipping on the 'skinny gene' The overall Sirt food diet is quite restrictive in terms of both food and calories, which can make it hard to stick too. There is still little reason to show that weight reduction is a more successful approach than any other diet regulated by calories.

In other terms, once you want to lose weight, why not consume things that you truly like consuming while becoming mindful of your daily consumption of calories?

Who should avoid the Sirt food diet?

Anyone who has diabetes wouldn't consider following the diet. And, if you're extremely successful, it might be hard to go if you go ahead, in the first stage of this plan, you might expect side effects such as headaches or light-headedness as your body adjusts according to the lower calorie intake.

The hype around Sirt food diet:

"Sirt food" sounds like something developed by aliens, brought to earth in the hopes of gaining control of mind and world domination for human consumption. Sirt foods contain molecules that shows Sirtuin-activating properties. Sirtuins are a form of protein that fruit flies and mice experiments have shown to control metabolism, improve muscle mass, and burn fat.

This program will help you lose fat and improve your strength, train your body for long-term success in weight loss, and a stronger, safer, and disease-free existence. All this as they enjoy red wine. It sounds like the dream meal, doesn't it? Ok, before you exhaust loading up on Sirtuin-activating ingredients from your investments, bear in mind the pros and cons.

How it works?

The secret to weight reduction is very easy at its core: either build a calorie deficit by raising your calorie consumption by exercise or reducing your calorie intake. So what if you can miss the diet and trigger a "skinny gene" without the need for an extreme calorie restriction instead? That is The Sirt food diet's premise. The way to do it is through Sirt foods.

Sirt foods are abundant in nutrients that activate a "skinny gene" named Sirtuin. The "skinny gene" is triggered when an energy deficiency is produced after the calories are limited. In 2003, Sirtuins became interesting to the world of nutrition when studies found that Resveratrol, a substance found in red wine, had the same impact on life period as calorie reduction but was accomplished without reducing intake.

The 39 members lost an average of seven pounds in seven days in the pilot study, evaluating the effectiveness of Sirtuins. Those results sound impressive but realizing this is a small sample size studied over a short time is important.

Weight-loss critics have concerns regarding the high predictions, too. The claims made are very speculative and extrapolate from studies mostly focused on the cellular level of simple organisms (like yeast). What is occurring at the molecular level does not automatically turn into what is occurring at the macro level within the human body.

What does the diet entail?

The diet is administered in two phases. Phase one lasts three days and reduces calories to 1,000 a day, consisting of three green juices and a meal approved for Sirt food. Step two lasts four days and decreases the average allotment by two green drinks and two meals to 1,500 calories each day.

There is a maintenance plan after these phases that is not focused on calories but on sensitive portions, well-balanced meals, and filling up on primarily Sirt foods.

The 14-day maintenance plan includes three meals, one green juice, and one or two snacks with Sirt food bites. Therefore followers are advised to perform 30 minutes of exercise five days a week.

Benefits of Sirt foods:

If you follow that diet closely, you will lose weight. Whether you are eating 1,000 calories of tacos, 1,000 calories of kale, or 1,000 calories of snickerdoodles, at 1,000 calories, you will lose weight. With a more sensible calorie reduction, you can achieve success. The average regular consumption of calories by those not on a diet is 2,000 to 2,200, but decreasing to 1,500 is also limiting and should be a successful weight-loss method for others.

Are there any precautions?

This strategy is strict with no wiggle room or substitutions, so weight control will only be achieved if the reduced calorie consumption is still sustained, rendering long-term commitment impossible.

That means that any weight you've lost in the first seven days will likely be gained back after you're done. Limiting the consumption of proteins with juices can contribute to loss of muscle mass. Losing muscle is synonymous with dropping your metabolic rate or 'metabolism' which makes it more difficult to maintain weight.

1.2 The Science of Sirtuins

Sirtuins are a protein family that controls cellular safety. Sirtuins are important in controlling cellular homeostasis. Homeostasis ensures that the cell is kept in order.

How Sirtuins Regulate Cellular Health with NAD+:

Think of the cells of the body as a workplace. There are several employees in the workplace employed on different projects for the common objective of remaining competitive and achieving the company's purpose for as long as possible in a productive manner. There are also many pieces in the cells that work on different tasks with the ultimate goal of staying healthy and functioning efficiently for as long as possible. Much as business goals shift regardless of different internal and external causes, so will cell goals. Someone must run the office, regulating what happens when who will do it and when to switch course. That would be your CEO in the office. They're the Sirtuins in the body at the cellular level.

Sirtuins a Protein Family:

Sirtuins consist of seven proteins that have a part to play in cell health. The Sirtuins can only function in the presence of NAD+, a coenzyme found in all living cells, nicotinamide adenine dinucleotide. NAD+ is essential to cellular metabolism and to hundreds of other processes in biology. It act as helper to cellular function.

Without it the body, cannot work. But NAD+ levels decrease with age, restricting Sirtuin activity even with age. It's not that simple, as all of the things in the human body. Sirtuins are controlling whatever occurs in the cells.

The Sirtuins are a protein family. Protein that sounds like nutritional protein — what's contained in beans and vegetables, and well, protein shakes — but in this case, we're thinking about molecules called proteins that act in a variety of different roles in the body's cells. Think of proteins as a company's teams, each focusing on their own particular task when collaborating with other divisions.

Hemoglobin is a well-known protein in the body, which is a member of the protein globin family, which is responsible for transporting oxygen in the blood. The myoglobin is the complement of the hemoglobin found in muscles, and together they comprise the family of globins.

Your body has about 60,000 protein families — a ton of departments — and one of those families is the Sirtuins. While hemoglobin is one of a two-protein band, Sirtuins are a 7-fold band.

Of the cell's seven Sirtuins, three work in the mitochondria, three work in the nucleus, and one works in the cytoplasm, each playing a variety of roles. However, the fundamental role of Sirtuins is to eliminate the acetyl groups from other proteins.

The specific reactions are controlled by acetyl groups. They're physical protein tags recognized by other proteins that will react with them. When proteins are the cell divisions and DNA is the Chairman, each department head's availability status is for the acetyl groups. For example, if a protein is accessible, then the Sirtuin will interact with it to make it possible, just like the Manager will collaborate with a department director accessible to get anything happening.

Sirtuins function for classes of acetyls by performing

what is called as deacetylation. This implies they know that on a molecule, there is an acetyl group and eliminate the acetyl group, which is teeing up the molecule for their work. One method by which Sirtuins work is by removing some specific biological proteins, such as histones, from the acetyl groups (deacetylating). Sirtuins, for example, deacetylate histones, proteins that form part of a condensed form of DNA called chromatin. The histone is a big, voluminous protein in which the DNA wraps itself. Consider it a Christmas tree, and the beach of DNA is the beach of lights. The chromatin is free or unwound when the histones have an acetyl ring.

This unwound chromatin means the transcription of the DNA, which is an essential process. But it doesn't need to stay unwound, because in this place it's prone to injury, much like the Christmas lights might get intertwined or the bulbs might get damaged because they're unwieldy or too long up. The chromatin is closed or firmly and conveniently wounded while the histones are deacetylated by Sirtuins, indicating gene expression is halted or silenced.

The History of Sirtuins:

In the 1970s, geneticist Dr. Amar Klar discovered the first Sirtuin, called SIR2, identifying it as a gene that controlled yeast cells' ability to match. Years later, in other organisms such as worms, fruit flies, other genes that were homologous were found by researchers—similar in structure — to SIR2, and these SIR2 homologs were then named Sirtuins. Every organism had a different number of Sirtuins. For e.g., yeast has five Sirtuins, one in bacteria, seven in mice, and seven homologs in humans from SIRT1 to SIRT7.

Experiments have been performed, and a trend has been

found, that the longest living strains of yeast have endured the best in the fridge, too.

That contributed to SIR2 being established as a gene that encouraged yeast longevity. Thus, the laboratory observed that eliminating SIR2 reduced yeast life span significantly, while, most notably, that the amount of SIR2 gene copies from one to two expanded the yeast life span. But, naturally, what activated SIR2 had yet to be found.

It is here that the acetyl groups come into play. Originally, it was believed that SIR2 might be a deacetylating enzyme — suggesting it separated certain acetyl groups — from other molecules, but nobody realized whether that was accurate, as all attempts to demonstrate that function in a test tube proved unsuccessful. In yeast, SIR2 could only deacetylate other proteins in the presence of the NAD+ coenzyme, nicotinamide adenine dinucleotide. SIR2 does little without NAD +. That was the critical finding of Sirtuin biology on the arc.

How Sirt foods help to burn fats?

Weight loss diet:

A scientific approach to battle weight gain follows the latest diet cleanse that has got the world raving about it.

The diet becomes common with the use of 'Sirt foods,' which are certain specific foods that function by stimulating somebody protein chains known as Sirtuins. According to science, these antioxidants act as protective agents that help slow the aging, boost the metabolism, and regulate the inflammation of the body, thereby helping in the loss of fat.

Studies have also indicated that the Sirt food diet can help people lose as much as seven pounds (3 kilos) in less than a week.

The menu allows you to have some of the most frequently available kitchen recipes and certain indulgent products as nuanced and logical as this diet plan looks. Some common foods that are permitted in this plan include foods such as oranges, dark chocolates, parsley, turmeric, kale, and even red.

The diet, though regarded a fad, focuses on maintaining a one-week strategy of restrictive weight loss. When you restrict your calorie consumption to 1000 kcal over the first three days (consuming three Sirt food green juices and eating a meal). You are permitted to raise your calorie intake to 1500kcal for the remaining days and have two meals a day (in addition to two Sirt food juices). Post this, and the maintenance process advises consuming two to three Sirtuin-rich, nutritious meals, combined with a successful weight-loss fitness routine, rendering it all the more manageable.

Since, in essence, it's restricting, others remain skeptical of the long-term diet program functioning. Your calorie intake is restricted by diet and can deprive you of other nutrients that are needed, so this is not a long-term, sustainable weight loss diet plan.

Instead of encouraging hunger and guilt over calorie intake, The Sirt food Diet is about using 'wonder foods' to turbocharge your body not only to increase weight loss but also to improve your overall health over the long term.

The research behind the diet is all about these Sirt foods, a collection of recently identified everyday plant foods rich in a chemical compound known as Sirtuin activators.

Such Sirtuin activators are a protein type that turns on the body's so-called 'skinny gene' pathways.

These skinny pathways are the same ones that are activated more commonly by fasting and exercise and help the body burn fat, increase muscle mass, and improve your health. Countries where people are now consuming a substantial amount of Sirt foods as part of their conventional diet, like Japan and Italy, are also consistently rated among the world's healthiest.

How it works?

Sirt foods stimulate Sirtuin genes, reportedly influencing the ability of the body to burn fat and boost the metabolic system.

Sirt food diet is two-stage based;

Stage One is a seven-day intensive program designed to kick-start your severe weight loss.

Then stage two is about upping the amount of Sirt food-rich products in your daily meals to keep weight loss.

Unlike several other short-term yo-yo plans, the Sirt food program provides recipes and guidance about how to hold away the weight you lose throughout the first week while trying to incorporate Sirt foods as part of a safe and balanced diet.

What to follow for staying on a Sirt food diet?

Stage One

Dieters drink two green juices a day for the first three days-including kale, celery, rocket, parsley, lemon, and green tea and eat one meal.

For example, with sage, chicken, and kale curry and prawn stir-fry with buckwheat noodles or sesame-glazed tofu, the meal may be something like turkey escalope, if you are vegetarian. Both made up of ingredients rich in Sirt food.

If you have cravings for sweets, you can also get 15-0.70 ounce of dark chocolate after your dinner.

You can consume two juices and two meals a day for the second half of your first week, with similar ingredients as for the first three days.

Stage Two

The focus shifts to eating 'normally' again after the initial stage of fasting, but upping your intake of the healthy Sirt foods.

There's a list of the top 30 foods rich in Sirtuins that sounds more like a trendy list of foods than a fresh, refined diet. Examples include arugula, chilies, coffee, green tea, dates of Medjool, red wine, turmeric, walnuts, and favorite health-conscious kale. Although the food that is being marketed as safe, it does not automatically encourage weight reduction on its own.

1.3 Top 30 Sirt foods to Lose weight

Red wine:

Red wine is produced by crushing and fermenting whole grapes of a dark color. Many forms of red wine range in flavor and color. Shiraz, Merlot, Cabernet Sauvignon, and Zinfandel are popular varieties. The amount of alcohol is typically between 12 and 15 percent. It has been shown that taking moderate amounts of red wine has health benefits. This is attributed largely to the high concentration of active antioxidants. Alcohol in wine is often believed to offer some of the advantages of low wine intake

Onions:

Onions are part of the plant family Allium, which also includes chives, garlic, and leeks. These vegetables have pungent taste characteristics and certain therapeutic properties.

The scale, form, color, and taste of the onions differ. The most common types of onions are red, yellow, and white. The flavor of these vegetables can vary from sweet and juicy to harsh, acidic, and pungent, sometimes based on the rising and consuming season.

Allium vegetables have been grown by farmers for generations. China is the world's largest producer of the onions. Chopping onions is common knowledge causing watery eyes. Yet onions will also offer possible health benefits. This may involve raising the likelihood of various forms of cancer, enhancing morale, and preserving good skin and hair.

Kale:

Kale is a nutrient-dense, black, leafy, cruciferous herb. It will offer a variety of health benefits for the whole body. It is a family member of the mustard, or Brassicaceae, as are the sprouts of cabbage and Brussels. Possible benefits include helping to manage blood pressure, boost digestive health, and cancer protection and type 2 diabetes.

Kale contains fiber, antioxidants, calcium, vitamins C and K, iron, and a wide variety of other nutrients that can help prevent various health issues. Antioxidants help the body eliminate undesirable toxins resulting from natural processes and environmental pressures. Such poisons are reactive compounds, known as free radicals. If too much build up in the body, they may cause harm to the cells. This can lead to health problems like inflammation and illnesses.

Soy:

Soy is a type of legume that is native to Asia. For thousands of years, soy has been part of traditional Asian diets. Today, soy is widely consumed, not only as a source of plant-based protein but as an ingredient in many processed foods too.

Soy is a healthy source of a few important nutrients.

Parsley:

Parsley is well known for being a flexible, new addition to sauces, salads, and any meal that can use a color pop and a bit of herbal flavor. Taken from the Petroselinum plant, parsley is a good source of many beneficial active ingredients, such as antioxidant flavonoids and phenolic compounds, as well as vitamin K, vitamin C, and beta-carotene vitamin A, a pigment that also gives the plant its vibrant tone. This herb also constitutes a great source of amino acid and folic acid, one of the most important vitamins of B.

Strawberries:

Fresh strawberries are among the most popular, nutritious, and refreshing fruits available. The soft, slightly tart berries have a strong antioxidant component and do not increase the blood sugar of a person easily, making them an excellent option for anyone with diabetes and healthy and tasty addition to any diet. All varieties of fruit and vegetables, including strawberries, provide several health benefits. Strawberries provide a host of possible benefits that may strengthen the body's protection against a number of diseases. There are more than 600 Strawberry types.

Extra virgin olive oil:

It is the unrefined oil you can buy and the highest quality olive oil. There are very specific standards that oil must meet to receive the "extra-virgin" label. Due to the way extra-virgin olive oil is produced, it retains the more true olive taste and has a lower oleic acid content than other olive oil varieties. It also incorporates many of the minerals and natural vitamins present in olives. Extra-virgin olive oil is identified as unrefined oil, as it is not treated with chemicals or temperature-changed.

What distinguishes it is the low oleic acid level and the absence of sensory flaws.

It contains no more than 1 percent oleic acid and is typically golden-green in color, with a specific flavor and a light peppery finish. Although you can cook with extra virgin olive oil, it has a lower smoke point than certain other oils, indicating it can burn at lower temperatures.

Dark chocolate (85% cocoa):

Dark chocolate is abundant in minerals, including copper, magnesium, zinc, etc. In dark chocolate, cocoa often includes antioxidants named flavonoids, which can have many benefits for the body. Chocolate comes from cacao, a plant that has a high mineral and antioxidant rates. Consumer milk chocolate is produced of cocoa butter, honey, cream, and tiny amounts of cacao. By comparison, dark chocolate contains even larger quantities of cacao and less sugar than chocolate with milk.

Buckwheat:

Buckwheat is in a group of foods commonly known as pseudocereals. Pseudocereals are seeds that are eaten as grains of cereals that do not grow on grasses. The quinoa and amaranth are also growing pseudocereals. Buckwheat is not linked to wheat despite its name and is thus gluten-free. It is used or refined into groats, rice, and noodles in buckwheat tea. The groats are the key ingredient in many popular European and Asian recipes, used in almost the same way as rice is. Buckwheat became popular as a health food because of its high content of minerals and antioxidants. Its benefits could include improved control of blood sugar.

Turmeric:

It is a spice that comes from the turmeric plant. Turmeric is commonly used for pain and inflammatory conditions, such as osteoarthritis.

This is often used for hay fever, insomnia, elevated cholesterol, a form of liver disorder, and scratching.

For heartburn, thinking and memory skills, inflammatory bowel disease, stress, and many other conditions, some people use turmeric, but there is no good scientific evidence to support these uses.

Walnuts:

Walnuts provide healthy vitamins, fats, fiber, and minerals — and that's just the beginning of how they can support your health. English walnut, which is also the most researched type, is the most common variety of walnut.

Matcha green tea:

Matcha is a form of green tea produced by taking young tea leaves into a bright green powder and grinding them to it. Then, the substance is whisked in the hot spray. That is distinct from traditional green tea, where the leaves are mixed with water and discarded afterward.

Arugula (rocket):

While arugula sometimes occurs in spring salad mixes, it is actually a part of the green cabbage and mustard family. This explains it's a signature peppery bite, much appreciated by chefs as well as home cooks. Also known as rocket, rucola, and roquette, the green can be found throughout the year but is in the early spring and fall peak season. It's simple and convenient to cook and nutritious, though it's more costly than plain old lettuce.

Lovage:

Lovage belongs to the parsley family used for gastrointestinal upsets, water accumulation, and skin disorders, and a digestive stimulant. The treatment of poor circulation and menstrual irregularities is also done by it.

Medjool dates:

Medjool dates are a range of dates enjoyed because of their natural sweetness. They are bigger, thicker, and taste more caramel-like than other traditional forms such as Deglet Noor. They are also sold dried but not dehydrated, rendering them soft and sticky. When they dry, their sugars get more intense, which further enhances their sweetness. Medjool dates are a concentrated, healthy nutrient source.

Bird's eye chili:

Birdeyechilis is a popular spice worldwide. Chilli peppers are sometimes used for cooking or cutting into salads, particularly in India and Asia. Birds Eyes are sometimes dried in shops. The red-orange chilies are packed in spice mills and have a clear shine. This freshly ground spice powder seems to be mainly sauced pungent for pungent amateur eaters.

Red chicory:

Red endive and red chicory have a bitter and pungent taste, mellowing when grilled or roasted. It is also ideal for adding flavor and zest to salads.

Capers:

The caper (Capparisspinosa or Capparisinermis) is the immature, unripened, green flower bud of the caper bush. Brined or dry, this caper is appreciated for the taste blast it brings to the dishes. It provides a large range of recipes of flavor and tanginess, including fish dishes, spaghetti, stews, and sauces.

Coffee:

Researchers confirmed results that coffee consumption is correlated with lower women's risk of depression, lower men's risk of lethal prostate cancer, and lower men's and women's risk for stroke.

Caffeine has been researched in coffee rather than any other component because the body part gained is the brain. It appears to get credit.

Blueberries:

Blueberries are wildly popular, sweet, nutritious, and. They've often labeled a superfood, low in calories, and incredibly good as highly nutrient-rich for you. They're so delicious and handy that they are considered by many as their favorite fruit.

Green Tea

The caffeine found in green tea acts as a stimulant, which has been shown in various studies to help fat burning and improve exercise performance. The massive range of antioxidants known as catechins helps to burn fat and boost the key to weight loss metabolism.

Apple

They say that one apple keeps the doctor away a day. In addition to being classified as a Sirt food, studies have shown that the fruit helps lower cholesterol and is a good source of fiber.

Salmon

Fatty fish like salmon are extremely nutritious and very rewarding, with very little calories leaving you complete for several hours. Salmon is filled with a protein of good quality, healthy fats, and numerous essential nutrients. Fish — and seafood in general — can also provide substantial iodine content. This nutrient is important for proper thyroid function, which is vital to optimally keep your metabolism running. Salmon is also a source of omega-3 fatty acids, which have been shown to help minimize inflammation, which is considered as a major factor in obesity and metabolic disease.

Boiled Potatoes

White potatoes, for some reason, seem to have fallen out of favor.

They do have several properties, however, which make them a perfect food — both for weight loss and optimal health.

They provide an amazingly wide variety of nutrients — a little of virtually all that you need.

For lengthy periods of time, there have even been accounts of people living on nothing but potatoes themselves.

They are particularly rich in potassium, a nutrient that most people don't get enough of, and that plays a significant role in controlling blood pressure.

White, boiled potatoes scored the highest out of all the foods on a scale called the Satiety Index, which measures how different satisfying foods are. What that means is that you'll probably feel satisfied and consume less of other things when consuming clean, boiled potatoes.

Tuna

Tuna is another food that is low in calories but has a high protein content.

It is a type of lean fish, which means it is small in calories.

Tuna is popular among gym freaks and fitness models on a break, as it's a perfect way to raise protein intake while retaining low total calories and fat content.

Soups

As already stated, low energy content meals and diets continue to help people consume fewer calories.

Most low-energy foods are those that contain much water, such as vegetables and fruits.

But you can only add water to your rice and create a soup.

Some experiments have found that consuming almost the same meal made into a broth rather than solid food helps people feel satiated and consume fewer calories substantially.

Apple Cider Vinegar

Apple cider vinegar is a popular item in the health-care community.

It is often used in condiments such as dressings or vinaigrettes and is even diluted in water by some people and drunk.

Some human-related experiments show that vinegar from apple cider can be helpful for weight reduction.

Adding vinegar to a high-carb meal can make people feel more full and eat 200–275 fewer calories for the rest of the day.

12-week research of obese adults also found that 0.5 to 1 ounce of vinegar a day induced 2.6–3.7 pounds to 1.2–1.7 kilograms of weight loss.

Chia Seeds

Chia seeds are perhaps the planet's most healthy crops.

They produce 12 grams of carbohydrates per ounce (0.98 ounces), which is relatively large, but the fiber is 11 of these grams.

This makes chia seeds a low-carbon diet and one of the world's greatest sources of fiber.

They can absorb at least 11–12 times their weight in

water, changing into a gel-like form and expanding in
your stomach because of its high fiber content.

1.4 Benefits of Sirt food Diet

There is growing proof that Sirtuin activators may have a wide variety of health benefits as well as muscle strengthening and appetite suppression. These include enhancing memory, helping the body better control blood sugar levels, and cleaning up the damage which results from free radical molecules that can accumulate in cells and lead to cancer and other conditions.

Strong observational evidence exists for the beneficial effects of Sirtuin-rich food and drinks intake in decreasing risks of chronic disease, said Professor Frank Hu, a Harvard University nutrition and epidemiology expert. A Sirt food diet is especially suited as an anti-aging regime.

Although activators of Sirtuin are found throughout the plant kingdom, only certain fruits and vegetables have sufficient quantities to count as Sirt foods. Examples include green tea, cocoa powder, turmeric for the Indian spice, kale, onions, and parsley.

Many of the fruits and vegetables on display in supermarkets, such as lettuce, tomatoes, avocados, bananas, carrots, kiwis, and cucumber, are actually rather low inactivators of Sirtuin. However, that doesn't imply they aren't worth consuming because they have plenty of other advantages.

The beauty of eating a Sirt food packed diet is that it's much more flexible than other diets. Simply adding some Sirt foods on top, you could eat healthily. Or you may be focused on getting them. The 5:2 diet could require more calories on low-calorie days, adding Sirt foods to claim.

One surprising result of a Sirt food diet trial is that participants lose substantial weight without sacrificing muscle. In fact, gaining muscle actually was common for participants, leading to a more defined and toned look.

That is Sirt foods' beauty; they activate fat burning, but they also enhance muscle growth, maintenance, and repair. This is completely opposite to other diets where weight loss typically comes from both fat and muscle, with muscle loss slowing down the metabolism and making it more likely to recover weight.

CHAPTER 02: EXERCISE, PHASES AND SAMPLE SIRT FOOD DIET PLAN

2.1 Building a Diet that works

Sirt foods are a recently discovered group of nutrient-rich foods that appear to be able to 'activate' the skinny genes of the body (also known as Sirtuins), in a way similar to fasting diets, with the same range of benefits, but without the common downsides of fasting diets, such as hunger, irritability and muscle loss.

By consuming a diet rich in Sirt foods, participants are believed to lose weight, build strength, look and sound better and maybe even lead a longer and safer life.

The Sirt food diet:

The nutritionists had developed the Sirt food Diet. They were so interested in Sirt foods' ability, and they developed a diet focused on optimizing the intake of Sirt food and minimal calories. They then tested this diet on exclusive London gym participants and were surprised by their findings. In the first seven days, gym participants dropped a total of 7lbs, despite not rising their workout rates. The participants not only shed a substantial amount of weight but also gained muscle (usually the reverse occurs while dieting) and reported significant improvements in overall health and well-being.

How the Sirt food diet actually work?

The diet is broken down into 2 phases. Phase 1: the 'hyper success phase' of 7 days, combining a Sirt food-rich diet with moderate calorie restriction, and Phase 2: the 'maintenance phase' of 14 days, where you consolidate your weight loss without limiting calories.

Is there any diet plan for the Sirt food diet?

Yes, there's a useful chart that tells you what you can eat every day, and when. The book includes all the recipes that you'll like for the first three weeks. There's a meat/fish option for every day and a vegetarian/vegan option. Nearly all of the recipes are gluten-free, and dairy-free options are available every day, meaning that this is a diet that will produce results for most people.

What happens after finishing the Sirt food diet?

The Sirt food Diet is not meant as a one-off 'diet' but instead as a way of life. You are encouraged to continue eating a diet rich in Sirt foods once you've completed the first three weeks and continue drinking your daily green juice. There's Sirt food Diet Recipe Chapter, with lots of more Sirt food-rich main meals, as well as recipes for alternatives to green juice and more hints and tips for following the Sirt food Diet. There are even some Sirt food dessert recipes. The phases 1 and 2 can be repeated as and when needed for a health boost, or if things have gone a little off course.

How to do the Sirt food plan?

The eating program describes the ingredients that turn on the so-called 'skinny genes' to increase metabolism and energy rates. It actually stipulates you may lose 7lbs in 7 days.

The eating plan will alter the way you eat healthily. It may sound like a name that is not user friendly, but it's one that you 're going to hear about a lot. Because the

'Sirt' is shorthand for the Sirtuin genes in Sirt foods, a group of genes nicknamed the 'skinny genes' that work, frankly, like magic.

Eating these foods, the plan's creators say, turns these genes on and mimics the effects of calorie limitation, fasting, and exercise. It activates a process of recycling in the body, clearing out the cellular debris and clutter that accumulates over time and causes ill health and vitality loss.

How diet works?

Sirt foods function by triggering the body's so-called "skinny gene" receptors, the same genes that are triggered while we are exercising or fast. This makes the body lose fat in a manner that mimics the limit on calories, even without the lack of nutrients or other shortages.

The sample of people studying the diet, including increased muscle mass and signs of feeling full and satisfied with food intake, reported an average loss of 7 pounds of weight in 7 days.

Sirt foods act as major regulators of our metabolism as a whole, most notably having effects on fat burning while at the same time increasing muscle and improving cellular fitness. Many of the foods falling into the Stir food category are often already associated with the world's healthiest diets-such as the typical Mediterranean diet. The program has two stages, with the first being the most intensive aspect of '7ibs-in-7-days' with the second going further at the side of things in terms of maintenance.

The special foods activate Sirtuins (SIRTs), a group of seven proteins found in the body which regulate the process of metabolism, inflammation, and aging. These particular proteins are known to protect cells against death due to stress. Researchers agree that Sirtuins often improve the body's ability to burn fat and raise metabolism. Certain plant compounds that increase the body's level of certain proteins. The Sirt food diet plan is based on around 20 foods including kale, red wine, onions, soy, strawberries, parsley, dark chocolate (85 percent cocoa), matcha green tea, extra virgin olive oil, buckwheat, turmeric, walnuts, coffee, arugula (rocket), bird's eye chili, lovage, Medjool dates, red chicory, blueberries, and capers.

The program claims eating certain foods would trigger your "skinny gene" course, and in seven days, you can lose seven pounds. Foods such as kale, dark chocolate, and wine contain a natural chemical called polyphenols, which mimic the effects of exercise and fasting. Strawberries, cinnamon, red onions, and turmeric are strong Sirt foods as well. The Sirtuin pathway can activate these foods to further cause weight loss. The science sounds enticing, but there is little research, in reality, to back up these claims. Plus, the expected weight loss pace in the first week is very high and not one or two pounds a week in accordance with the National Institute of Health 's recommendations on healthy weight loss.

The diet has two phases:

2.2 Phase One of Sirt food Diet

It will last for seven days. You'll consume three Sirt food green juices and one Sirt food-rich meal for a minimum of 1,000 calories over the first three days. You consume two green beverages and two meals on days four and seven, for a minimum of 1,500 calories.

The first process lasts for seven days, with calorie restriction and plenty of green juice included. It's supposed to improve your weight reduction and promises to help you drop 7 pounds (3.2 kg) in seven days.

The intake of calories during the first three days of phase one is limited to 1,000 calories. You consume three green drinks, plus one meal, every day. You will select from recipes in the book every day, many of which include Sirt food as a big part of the meal.

Examples of meals include miso-glazed tofu, the omelet Sirt food, or a shrimp stir-fry with buckwheat noodles.

Calorie consumption is raised to 1,500 on days 4–7 of step one. This involves two green juices a day and two more Sirt food-rich meals that can be picked from the guide.

2.3 Phase Two of Sirt food Diet

It is a 14-day maintenance plan, although it is designed to keep you losing weight (not keeping your current weight). Each day is comprised of three healthy Sirt foods and green tea.

You're urged to start consuming a Sirt-rich diet and drinking a green juice every day during these three weeks. Various Sirt food cookbooks and recipes can be found online on the Sirt food website. One green juice recipe found on the Sirt food website includes a combination of kale and other leafy greens, parsley, celery, green apple, ginger, lemon juice, and matcha. Buckwheat and lovage are also recommended ingredients for the use of your green juice. The diet advises producing juices in a juicer, not a blender, because it tastes healthier.

Step two requires two weeks to finish. You should continue to lose weight steadily during this "maintenance" phase.

This step has no clear calorie limit. Instead, you eat three Sirt food meals and one green juice a day. The meals are again picked from the recipes included in the book.

The possible cost of Sirt food diet:

You really have to plan and have access to the recommended ingredients to follow that diet properly. You'll need to invest in a proper juicer too, which will run you at least $100.

The seasonality of products makes having strawberries and kale a little difficult at some periods of the year. Following on while traveling, at social gatherings, and feeding a family containing small children is sometimes tough.

The diet itself leaves off multiple food classes and is restrictive. Dairy products are not included on the menu, which provides an abundance of important nutrients and some that most people lack. Furthermore, the polyphenol-rich food matcha often contains lead in the tea leaves, which, especially when taken regularly, is potentially dangerous to your health. Like 85 percent dark chocolate, it also has a strong and bitter flavor, which is also recommended.

Surely, polyphenol-rich foods can be included in a weight loss plan, but they are not the basis for a whole diet. Of course, you don't need everyday wine and dark chocolate, plus too much matcha is potentially dangerous.

2.4 Exercise along with diet

Pilates is a mind-body workout, with every exercise targeting your core muscles. Whether you're targeting other muscles or making a core-focused move, during a Pilates session, your core is always engaging. And the workout method will strengthen all of your core areas. "To gain true core power, the abdominal [area] operates on both the deep and superficial stages.

Leg Circle

• Lie face up by your hands on your sides, palms flat.

• Bend your left knee and put the left foot flat on the floor. Extend your right leg, so it is perpendicular to the ground.

• Circle your right leg sideways, down to the ground, and return to the starting position. You can make the round as large as you can while retaining your bottom back on the floor.

• Overturn the circle.

• Complete all reps with one leg, then replicate with the other.

The One Hundred

• Lie with your face up.

• Raise the two legs up to the ceiling and drop them partially until they are bent.

• Twist your head backward and stretch your arms alongside your body with palms downwards.

• Pump up and down your arms as you inhale five counts, and exhale five counts.

• Repeat ten times the breathing rhythm while

maintaining the pose.

Single-Leg Stretch

• Lie with your Face-up.

• Touch your chest with both of your knees, put your hands on your shins, and curl your head up off the floor.

• Stretch out one leg at a time, alternating sides.

• Keep your lower back on the floor while keeping your core engaged.

Criss-Cross

• Lie face-up and put both of your knees in your chest.

• Place your hands behind your head and hold your elbows broad. Curl your head upwards.

• Put your left shoulder to your right knee while stretching your left leg. Bring your right elbow against your left knee while you stick out your right hip.

• Continue switching sides.

Double Leg Stretch

• Lie face-up and put both of your knees towards your chest. Curl your head up and put hands n knees.

• Spread out both legs in front of you when you raise your arms overhead. Try to keep your legs as straight as you can while keeping your bottom on the floor.

• Cross your arms out and around back to your knees as you draw back your knees to the chest.

Scissor Kick

• Lie with face up.

• Stretch the right leg until it's perpendicular to the

ground. Place your hands to your right leg, bring it to your chest, and curl up your head. Pick the left leg a few centimeters off the surface.

• Switch the legs, pull the left leg in toward you and let the right leg hover over the floor.

• Continue to switch legs.

Teaser

• Lie with your Face-up. Bend knees over your hips, and lift your foot from the ground.

• Stretch your legs as you reach your arms towards feet and raise your head and shoulders off the ground. Seek to bring the torso and legs into a V formation.

• Hold for 5 seconds, and then bend your knees sideways by rolling on your back.

Pendulum

• Lie face-up with arms held out on the sides. Bend knees over your hips, and lift your foot from the ground.

• Raise your knees to the right, holding the butt down on the ground.

• Return to the beginning, then repeat on the other leg.

Plank Leg Lift

• Start with your hands directly beneath your shoulders on a high plank.

• Alternate lifting one leg as high as you can from the floor but not past shoulder level.

• Keep the core, ass, and quads involved to avoid hip rocking.

Plank Rock

• Start with your hands directly beneath your shoulders on a high plank.

• Rock your whole body forward a couple of inches toward your hands and then back toward your heels.

• Keep the core, the ass, and the quads engaged all the time.

Slow Motion Mountain Climber

• Start with your hands immediately under your shoulders on a high plank.

• Take one knee up at a time to the chest.

• Hold the core, butt, and quads engaged in stopping hip rocking.

Hip Dip

• Start with your right hand right under your right shoulder on a sideboard and your left foot stacked on top of the right.

• Dip your hips towards the ground, then lift them up again.

• Repeat ten times before turning to left-hand.

2.5 Sample Sirt food Diet Plan

Day: 1

Breakfast: Kale, edamame and tofu curry

Snack: The Sirt food Juice

Lunch: Honey, garlic and Chilli oven-roasted Squash

Dinner: Grape and melon juice

Day: 2

Breakfast: Kale and blackcurrant smoothie

Snack: Summer Berry Smoothie

Lunch: Homemade Roasted Celery Hummus

Dinner: Ginger Turmeric Lemonade

Day: 3

Breakfast: Chocolate berry smoothie

Snack: **Green Tea Smoothie**

Lunch: baked potatoes with spicy chickpea stew

Dinner: Grape and melon juice

Day: 4

Breakfast: Sirt food breakfast Scramble

Snack: Ginger Turmeric Lemonade

Lunch: Pizza Kale Chips

Dinner: Kale, edamame and tofu curry

Day: 5

Breakfast: Smoked Salmon Omelet

Snack: Summer Berry Smoothie

Lunch: Turmeric baked salmon

Dinner: Grape and melon juice

Day: 6

Breakfast: Mushroom Scramble Eggs

Snack: The Sirt food Juice

Lunch: Asian king prawn

Dinner: **Green Tea Smoothie**

Day: 7

Breakfast: Mushroom Buckwheat Pancakes

Snack: Kale and blackcurrant smoothie

Lunch: Turmeric baked salmon

Dinner: Summer Berry Smoothie

CHAPTER 03: GROCERY LIST AND SIRT FOOD DIET RECIPES (50 RECIPES)

3.1 List of Foods to Buy

Red wine

Onions

Kale

Soy

Parsley

Strawberries

Extra virgin olive oil

Dark chocolate (85% cocoa)

Buckwheat

Turmeric

Walnuts

Matcha green tea

Arugula (rocket)

Lovage

Medjool dates

Bird's eye chili

Red chicory

Capers

Coffee

Blueberries

3.2 Recipes for Breakfast

1) Sirt food breakfast Scramble

Ingredients:

0.166 ounce mild curry powder

½ bird's eye chili, thinly sliced

2 eggs

0.166 ounce ground turmeric

A handful of thinly sliced mushrooms

Take 0.17 ounce parsley, finely chopped

Add a seed mixture for topping and some Rooster Sauce for flavor

0.70 ounce kale, roughly chopped

0.166 ounce extra virgin olive oil

Instructions:

Mix the curry and turmeric powder, then apply a little water until a soft paste has been produced.

Steam up the kale for 2-3 minutes.

Use medium heat to warm oil in a frying pan and fry the chili and mushrooms for 2-3 minutes before they start browning and softening.

Add the eggs and spice paste, and cook over medium heat, then add the kale and continue cooking for another minute over medium heat. Attach the parsley, then blend well and enjoy.

2) Summer Berry Smoothie

Ingredients:

14 ounce frozen mixed berries

6 ounce vanilla Greek yogurt

0.5 ounce honey optional

14 ounce apple juice can also use almond milk, skim milk, coconut milk or another flavor of the Juice

One banana sliced

Optional garnish: fresh berries and mint sprigs

Instructions:

In a blender, put the apple juice, banana, berries, and yogurt; blend until smooth. If you think the texture of the smoothie is too thick, add the liquid (1/4 cup) a bit more.

Taste and, if desired, add the honey. Do a topping of fresh berries and mint sprigs if needed, then squeeze into two cups.

3) Rocket and Arugula Salad

Ingredients:

1.4 ounce rocket leaves

1 ounce red wine

Salt as required

8 ounce arugula

2.8 ounce pear

0.35 ounce toasted walnuts

0.35 ounce yogurt (curd)

Powdered black pepper as required

Dressing:

0.43 ounce virgin olive oil

1 ounce of lemon juice

1 ounce balsamic vinegar

Instructions:

Wash the pears, remove and break them into thin pieces under running water. Soak them up and cool them in a medium bowl filled with red wine.

Whisk balsamic vinegar, pure olive oil, and lemon juice together in a bowl to make the dressing for the salad. With this dressing, toss the rocket and arugula in a medium bowl and sprinkle salt and black pepper powder over the leaves.

Put the poached pears nicely around the salad and top with yogurt and toasted walnuts.

4) Chocolate Berry Smoothie

Ingredients:

0.5 ounce chia seeds

0.33 ounce cocoa powder or cacao

Add 250 ml (8 ounce) milk of your choice

One very ripe banana

0.5 ounce maple syrup

Add 3.52 ounce (3/4 cup) mixed frozen berries (I use a mix of blackberries, raspberries, blackcurrants, and redcurrants)

Instructions:

Place in a blender and scramble all the ingredients until smooth. Pour into a glass, then serve.

5) Smoked Salmon Omelet

Ingredients:

2 Medium eggs

3.52 ounce Smoked salmon, sliced

0.083 ounce Capers

10 g Rocket, chopped

0.166 ounce Parsley, chopped

0.166 ounce Extra virgin olive oil

Instructions:

Crack eggs into a bowl. Add the tuna, capers, parsley, and shot.

In a non-stick frying pan, fire up the olive oil until

heated but not smoking. Add the egg mixture and move the mixture around the pan, using a spatula or fish slice until it is even. Reduce heat, and let it cook through the omelet.

Insert the spatula around the edges and roll the omelet up or fold in half to serve.

6) Apple Pancakes with Blackcurrant Compote

Ingredients:

2.64 ounce porridge oats

4.40 ounce plain flour

1 ounce caster sugar

Pinch of salt

0.166 ounce baking powder

Take-Two apples then peel them and cut into small pieces

300ml partially skimmed milk

2 egg whites

0.33 ounce light olive oil

For the compote:

4.23 ounce blackcurrants washed and stalks removed

1 ounce caster sugar

3 tbsp water

Instructions:

Make the compote first. Transfer the blackcurrants, water, and sugar in a saucepan. Bring to a cooker and simmer for 10-15 minutes.

In a big pot, combine the oats, flour, baking powder, caster sugar, and salt and blend well. Stir in the apple and whisk a little at a time in the milk before you have a smooth mix. Whisk the egg whites then insert into the flour for the pancake. Bring the batter over to a tub.

Heat 0.083 ounce of oil over medium-high heat in a non-stick frying pan and add approximately one-quarter of the batter. Cook until light brown, on all hands. Remove for four pancakes and repeat to produce.

Eat the pancakes drizzled over with blackcurrant compote.

7) Mushroom Scramble Eggs

Ingredients:

Take two eggs

0.166 ounce ground turmeric

0.70 ounce kale, roughly chopped

0.166 ounce extra virgin olive oil

0.166 ounce mild curry powder

½ bird's eye chili, thinly sliced

Take a handful of button mushrooms, thinly sliced

0.17 ounce parsley, finely chopped

Add a seed mixture as a topping and some Rooster Sauce for flavor

Instructions:

Mix the curry and turmeric powder and apply some water until a soft paste has been obtained.

Steam up the kale 2–3 minutes.

Use medium heat to warm the oil in a frying pan and cook the chili and mushrooms for 2–3 minutes before browning and softening has started.

8) Mushroom Buckwheat Pancakes

Ingredients:

1.94 ounce wholemeal flour

1.94 ounce buckwheat flour

9 ounce Alpro Almond Milk

One free-range egg

1.05 ounce butter, for frying

For the filling:

1.76 ounce flour

1.76 ounce butter

9 ounce Alpro Almond Milk

One free-range egg3.52 ounce sliced chestnut mushrooms

Three large handfuls of baby spinach

Olive oil

9 ounce Alpro Almond Milk

One free-range egg

Instructions:

Melt butter in a saucepan 1.76 ounce. Use the flour to create a paste. Continue cooking for 30 seconds.

Gradually add the milk, stirring vigorously until the white sauce is smooth. (Make sure to stir well so that lumps do not form.)

Fry the mushrooms in the oil until the spinach is brown and wilt. Drop the mushrooms into the white sauce, add the cheese and nutmeg to taste, then season.

In the meantime, add the two flour types to a bowl, and make a small well.

Whisk the egg into the milk, lightly. Pour a handful of the egg mixture into the flour and continue whisking. Start applying the liquid and whisking until the batter is smooth.

Melt the butter and add a ladle of the batter in a non-stick frying pan. Swirl to brush the base of the pan equally, then turn it as the pancake is shakeable. Repeat until all the batter has been consumed, and then line it with mushroom and spinach stuffing.

9) Sirt Muesli

Ingredients:

0.70 ounce buckwheat flakes

0.52 ounce coconut flakes or desiccated coconut

1.41 ounce Medjool dates, pitted and chopped

0.35 ounce buckwheat puffs

0.52 ounce walnuts, chopped

0.35 ounce cocoa nibs

3.52 ounce plain Greek yogurt (or vegan alternative, such as soya or coconut yogurt)

3.52 ounce strawberries, hulled and chopped

Instructions:

Mix all of the mentioned ingredients together (Add strawberries and yogurt later if not eating right away)

10) Choc Chip Granola

Ingredients:

7.05 ounce jumbo oats

1.76 ounce pecans, roughly chopped

3 tbsp light olive oil

0.70 ounce butter

0.5 ounce dark brown sugar

1 ounce rice malt syrup

2.11 ounce good-quality (70%)

dark chocolate chips

Instructions:

Oven preheated to 320°F (284°F fan / Gas 3). Line a large baking tray with a sheet of silicone or parchment for baking.

In a wide dish, add the oats and the pecans. Steam the olive oil, butter, brown sugar, and rice malt syrup gently in a medium non-stick pan before the butter has melted and the sugar and syrup dissolved. Do not let simmer. Pour the syrup over the oats and mix vigorously until completely coated with the oats.

Scatter the granola over the baking tray and push out through the corners. Leave water clumps with mixing, instead of just scattering. Bake for 20 minutes in the oven until golden brown is only tinged at the edges. Remove from the oven, and leave completely to cool on the tray.

When it is cool, break with your fingers any larger lumps on the tray and then mix in the chocolate chips.

Place the granola in an airtight tub or pot, or spill it. The granola is to last for at least two weeks.

11) Lentil Soup

Ingredients:

Four garlic cloves, pressed or minced

2 teaspoons ground cumin

0.166 ounce curry powder

¼ cup extra virgin olive oil

One medium yellow or white onion, chopped

Two carrots, peeled and chopped

½ teaspoon dried thyme

Take one large can (28 ounces) diced tomatoes, lightly drained

Add 8 ounce brown or green lentils, picked over and rinsed

Take Freshly ground black pepper, to taste

Add 8 ounce chopped fresh collard greens or kale, tough ribs removed

Add 1 to 1 ounce lemon juice (½ to 1 medium lemon), to taste

4 cups vegetable broth

2 cups of water

0.166 ounce salt, more to taste

Pinch of red pepper flakes

Instructions:

Heat the olive oil over medium heat in a large Dutch

oven or pot. One-fourth cup olive oil may sound like a lot, but this nutritious soup adds a beautiful richness and heart to it.

Add the chopped onion and carrot and cook, frequently stirring, until the onion has softened and turns translucent, about 5 minutes after the oil has shimmered.

Add the garlic, cumin, thyme and curry powder. Cook for about 30 seconds, while constantly stirring, until fragrant. Pour in the drained diced tomatoes and cook for another few minutes, stirring regularly to improve their flavor.

Garnish with lentils, broth, and rice. Add a pinch of red pepper flakes and 0.166 ounce salt. Season generously with black pepper, newly soiled. Raise heat and bring the mixture to a boil, then partially cover the pot and lower heat to keep a mild simmer—Cook for 25 to 30 minutes, or until the lentils are tender but keep their shape still.

Transfer 2 soup cups to a blender. Fasten the lid securely, protect your hand against steam with a tea towel placed over the lid, and purée the soup until smooth. Pour the puréed soup back into the saucepan. (Or, to mix a part of the soup using an immersion blender.)

Attach the chopped greens and cook for an additional 5 minutes, or until the greens soften to your taste. Remove the pot from heat, and stir in 1 lemon juice tablespoon. Taste and add more salt, pepper and/or lemon juice to the season until the flavors sing. Add another pinch or two red pepper flakes for spicier soup.

Serve while you're hot. Leftovers are kept in the refrigerator for about four days, or can be frozen for several months (just defrosting before serving).

12) Strawberry Buckwheat Tabbouleh

Ingredients:

1⁄3 cup (1.76 ounce) buckwheat

0.5 ounce ground turmeric

1⁄2 cup (80g) avocado

3⁄8 cup (65g) tomato

1⁄8 cup (0.70 ounce) red onion

1⁄8 cup (25g) Medjool dates, pitted

0.5 ounce capers

3⁄4 cup (1.05 ounce) parsley

2⁄3 cup (3.52 ounce) strawberries, hulled

0.5 ounce extra virgin olive oil

juice of 1⁄2 lemon

1 ounce (1.05 ounce) arugula

Instructions:

Cook the buckwheat with the turmeric as directed on the package.

Drain to cool, and set aside.

Chop the avocado, dates, tomato, red onion, capers, and parsley thinly and combine with the cool buckwheat.

Break the strawberries, then blend the oil then lemon juice softly into the salad. Serve on arugula of bed.

13) Vegetable and Nut Loaf

Ingredients:

One onion, medium chopped

0.166 ounce dried thyme

0.166 ounce dried marjoram

0.166 ounce dried basil

0.166 ounce dried tarragon

0.5 ounce butter or oil

2 cups finely chopped mushrooms

Two cloves garlic, finely chopped

0.166 ounce dried sage

Red wine or sherry

Take 8 ounce cottage cheese

Add 3/4 pound grated cheese: Parmesan, Gruyere, cheddar, fontina, smoked or any combination

Add 4 ounce mixed fresh chopped herbs such as parsley, oregano, thyme

Add salt and pepper

Add 2 cups cooked brown rice

Add 2 cups walnuts, finely chopped or pulsed in a food processor

Add 8 ounce cashews or almonds, finely chopped or pulsed in a food processor

Five eggs

Instructions:

Preheat oven to 350°F.

In oil or butter, whisk in the onion until it starts to melt. Remove the mushrooms and a tablespoon of salt and pepper, then simmer before the mushrooms detach then soften their juices. Mix the garlic and dried herbs, then start cooking. If the pan starts drying out again, apply a decent splash of red wine or sherry and simmer before it gets smaller. The products should be damp, but they do not float in the oil. Allow cooling for a bit by turning the heat off.

While the mushroom mix cools a 9-inch loaf pan and line with parchment paper or foil, butter or oil cools down.

Add the brown rice and nuts together in a large bowl. The eggs with the cottage cheese were beaten in a separate bowl. Attach the egg mixture to the mixture of rice and nut, then whisk in the cooled mushrooms, grated cheese, and fresh herbs. Blend well. Taste to adapt and season. (You should cook up a little patty to try if you're concerned about the raw egg)

You can store the mixture sealed in the fridge for no more than a day.

Cover the loaf pan with the mixture of nuts, rap on the counter a few times to prevent any air bubbles, and clean the rim with a spatula. Decorate with mushroom slices, bell pepper slices, or entire walnuts, if needed. Put the loaf pan into a baking tray.

Bake until the loaf is firm for about an hour (slightly longer when the mixture is cooled). Remove from the frying pan. Rest on a cooling stand for ten minutes, then use the excess parchment paper or foil to extract the loaf out of the pan. Peel the parchment or foil and serve garnished with new herbs on a platter.

Serve with your favorite autumn vegetables accompanied by a mushroom gravy.

3.3 Recipes for Lunch

14) Honey, garlic and Chilli oven-roasted Squash

Ingredients:

1 kg assorted squash and pumpkin (at least five different types), cut in medium size pieces

3 Tbsp (15 ml) olive oil

Three whole garlic cloves, lightly crushed

Four red or green chilies, slit down the middle

2 sprigs thyme

3 Tbsp (15 ml) honey

One sprig rosemary

Salt and pepper to taste

Instructions:

Preheat the oven to 300°F.

Take a large bowl and add al the ingredients and allow to stand for 30 minutes, mixing occasionally.

In a roasting tray, place the Squash and cover with foil.

Roast covered at 300°F for 10 minutes.

Increase the temperature of the oven to 350°F, remove the foil, and roast for another 10 minutes to allow the Squash to caramel lightly.

15) Homemade Roasted Celery Hummus

Ingredients:

One green serrano chili, minced (optional)

8 ounce cooked chickpeas

1/3 cup tahini

1 ouncefresh lime or lemon juice

Four stalks of celery, trimmed and cut into 1 cm pieces (about 8 ounce)

Five tablespoons olive oil (preferably EV)

2 pods of garlic

0.166 ounce salt or to taste

0.5 ounce minced parsley

Instructions:

Place the celery into a baking platter.

Top with two spoonfuls of oil

Place the two garlic pods in a plate corner, and scatter with the chili.

Bake at 350°F for 45 minutes in an oven.

Put the chickpeas into the mixer.

Carry some remaining oil into the mixer, in the hot roasted celery and other vegetables.

Add tahini, lime or lemon juice, salt, and mix until light and smooth for 3-4 minutes.

Remove from the blender into a bowl, add the remaining 1.5 ounce of olive oil and chopped parsley.

16) Pizza Kale Chips

Ingredients:

0.166 ounce dried Oregano

0.166 ounce dried Marjoram

0.166 ounce Garlic Powder

0.166 ounce Onion Powder

8 cup Kale, leaves from about six stalks, veins removed

8 ounce raw Cashews

4 ounce Tomato Paste, one small can

1 ounce Nutritional Yeast, Lewis Labs Brewers Yeast Buds (from sugar beets)

0.083 ounce Salt

1/4 tsp Red Pepper Flakes

0.166 ounce dried Basil

0.083 ounce dried Rosemary

Instructions:

Place the cashews in a tub, cover with filtered water and allow the cashews, preferably overnight, to soak refrigerated for at least 2 hours.

Drain away the cashew juice. Place the cashews in a meal processor or blender. To only cover the cashews, apply filtered water, and heat until creamy smooth.

Stir together the cashew cream in a large mixing bowl with all remaining ingredients except the kale. Stir until the combination is even.

Rinse the kale and take the leaves off the fibrous roots. Tear the pieces into "chip" size.

Take the kale away with the cashew cream filled with

"pizza." You may need to do this a little bit at a time, making sure that coverage is assured.

Dehydrate the kale chips for 12 hours, then cook at 105-115°F.

17) Asian king prawn

Ingredients:

5.29 ounce shelled raw king prawns, deveined

2 tsp extra virgin olive oil

2.64 ounce soba (buckwheat noodles)

Add 2 tsp of tamari

One garlic clove, finely chopped

One bird's eye chili, finely chopped

0.70 ounce red onions, sliced

1.41 ounce celery, trimmed and sliced

2.64 ounce green beans, chopped

0.166 ounce finely chopped fresh ginger

3.38 ounce chicken stock

0.17 ounce lovage or celery leaves

1.76 ounce kale, roughly chopped

Instructions:

Heat a frying pan over a high flame, then cook the prawns for 2-3 minutes in 1 teaspoon tamari and 0.166 ounce oil. Load the prawns into a tray. Wipe the pan out with paper from the kitchen, because you would be using it again.

Cook the noodles for 5-8 minutes in boiling water, or as

directed on the packet. Drain and put away.

Meanwhile, over medium-high heat, fry the garlic, Chilli and ginger, red onion, celery, beans, and kale in the remaining oil for 2-3 minutes. Attach the stock and bring to the boil, then simmer for one to two minutes until the vegetables are cooked but crunchy.

Attach the prawns, noodles, and leaves of lovage/celery to the oven put back to the boil, then reduce from the heat and serve.

18) Turmeric baked salmon

Ingredients:

4.4 -5.29 ounce Skinned Salmon

0.166 ounce Extra virgin olive oil

0.166 ounce ground turmeric

1/4 Juice of a lemon

For the spicy celery

0.166 ounce Extra virgin olive oil

1.4 ounce Red onion, finely chopped

2.11 ounce Tinned green lentils

1 Garlic clove, finely chopped

1 cm fresh ginger, finely chopped

1 Bird's eye chili, finely chopped

5.29 ounce Celery, cut into 2cm lengths

0.166 ounce Mild curry powder

4.58 ounce Tomato, cut into eight wedges

3.38 ounce Chicken or vegetable stock

0.5 ounce Chopped parsley

Instructions:

Heat the oven to 390°F.

Start with the sparkling celery. Heat over medium-low heat a frying pan, add olive oil, then onion, garlic, ginger, chili, and celery. Fry for at least three minutes or until softened but not colored, then add the curry powder and cook for a minute further.

Then add the tomatoes, stock, and lentils and gently simmer for 10 minutes. Depending on how crispy you like your celery, you might want to increase or decrease the cooking time.

In the meantime, mix together the turmeric, oil, and lemon juice and rub over the salmon.

Transform into a baking tray and cook for 8–10 minutes.

Stir the parsley through the celery to finish, and serve with salmon.

19) Baked potatoes with spicy chickpea stew

Ingredients:

4-6 baking potatoes, pricked all over

1 ounces olive oil

Four cloves garlic, grated or crushed

2cm ginger, grated

Two red onions, finely chopped

½ -2 teaspoons chili flakes (depending on how hot you like things)

1 ounce cumin seeds

2 tablespoons turmeric

Splash of water

2 x 14-ounce tins chopped tomatoes

1 ounce unsweetened cocoa powder (or cacao)

2 x 14-ounce tins chickpeas (or kidney beans if you prefer) including the chickpea water DON'T DRAIN!!

Two yellow peppers (or whatever color you prefer!), chopped into bite size pieces

1 ounce parsley plus extra for garnish

Salt and pepper to taste (optional)

Side salad (optional)

Instructions:

Preheat the oven to 390°F while you can prepare all the supplies you need.

Put your baking potatoes in the oven when the oven is hot enough, and cook them for 1 hour or until as long as they are done as you like them.

Add the olive oil and chopped red onion in a large wide saucepan once the potatoes are in the oven and cook gently with the lid until the onions are soft but not brown for 5 minutes.

Remove the lid and add the garlic, cumin, ginger, and Chilli. Cook on low heat for another minute, then add the turmeric and a few drops of water and cook for another minute, being careful not to let the saucepan get too hot.

Add cocoa (or cacao) powder, chickpeas (including chickpea water), and yellow pepper in the tomatoes. Put to boil and cook for 45 minutes at low heat until the sauce is heavy and unctuous (but don't let it burn!). The stew should be handled at the same time as the potatoes.

At last, stir in the 1 ounce of parsley and some salt and pepper, if desired, and serve the stew over the baked potatoes, perhaps with a simple side salad.

20) Chinese-Style pork with pak choi

Ingredients:

14 ounce firm tofu, cut into large cubes

0.5 ounce corn flour

0.5 ounce water

125ml chicken stock

0.5 ounce rice wine

0.5 ounce tomato puré

0.166 ounce brown sugar

0.5 ounce soy sauce

One clove garlic, peeled and crushed

One thumb (5cm) fresh ginger, peeled and grated 0.5 ounce rapeseed oil

3.52 ounce shiitake mushrooms, sliced

One shallot, peeled and sliced

Take 7.05 ounce pak choi or Choi sum, cut into thin slices 14 ounce pork mince (10% fat)

3.52 ounce bean sprouts

Large handful (0.70 ounce) parsley, chopped.

Instructions:

Put the Tofu on paper for the kitchen, cover with more

paper for the kitchen, and set aside.

Mix the water and corn flour together in a small bowl, removing all the lumps. Add the chicken stock, rice wine, purée tomatoes, brown sugar, and sauce soya. Attach the smashed garlic and ginger, then mix.

Add oil and heat to a high temperature in a wok or wide frying pan. Attach the shiitake mushrooms, then stir-fry until cooked, then shiny for 2–3 minutes. Yake mushrooms out pf the pan and put aside with a slotted spoon. Attach the Tofu to the saucepan and stir-fry both sides until golden. Remove with a spoon and set aside.

Add the shallot and Choi mixture to the wok, stir-fry for 2 minutes, then apply the thinner. Cook until the slim is cooked through, then add the sauce, reduce a notch of heat. Attach the beansprouts, mushrooms shiitake, and Tofu to the saucepan and cook up. Remove from oil, whisk in the parsley, and immediately serve.

21) Tuscan Bean Stew

Ingredients:

0.5 ounce extra virgin olive oil

1.76 ounce red onion, finely chopped

1.05 ounce carrot, peeled and finely chopped

1.05 ounce celery, trimmed and finely chopped

One garlic clove, finely chopped

½ bird's eye chili, finely chopped (optional)

0.166 ounce herbes de Provence

6.76 ounce vegetable stock

1 x 14 ounce tin chopped Italian tomatoes

0.166 ounce tomato purée

7.05 ounce tinned mixed beans

1.76 ounce kale, roughly chopped

0.5 ounce roughly chopped parsley

1.41 ounce buckwheat

Instructions:

Put the oil over low to medium heat in a medium saucepan and fry the onion, carrot, celery, garlic, chili, and herbs gently until the onion is soft but not colored.

Stir in stock, tomatoes, and purée tomatoes and carry to boil. Attach the beans and require to cook for 30 minutes.

Cook for another 5-10 minutes after adding kale, then add the parsley until tender.

In the meantime, cook the buckwheat as instructed by the package, drain and then serve with stew.

22) Kale and red onion dhal with buckwheat

Ingredients:

0.5 ounce olive oil

One small red onion, sliced

Three garlic cloves, grated or crushed

2 cm ginger, grated

2 teaspoons turmeric

2 teaspoons garam masala

5.64 ounce red lentils

400ml coconut milk

6.76 ounce water

One birds eye chili, deseeded and finely chopped

3.52 ounce kale (spinach can also be used)

5.64 ounce buckwheat (or brown rice)

Instructions:

In a big, deep saucepan, place the olive oil and add the sliced onion. Cook at low pressure, with the cover on until softened for 5 minutes.

Add the garlic, Chilli, and ginger and cook for 1 minute.

Add the turmeric, garam masala, sprinkle with water, and cook for 1 minute.

Add the red lentils, coconut milk, and 200 ml of water (simply fill the coconut milk with water and tap it into the casserole).

23) Char grilled beef with onion rings, garlic kale and herb roasted potatoes.

Ingredients:

3.5-ounce potatoes, peeled and cut into 2cm dice

0.5 ounce extra virgin olive oil

0.17 ounce parsley, finely chopped

1.76 ounce red onion, sliced into rings

1.76 ounce kale, sliced

One garlic clove, finely chopped

5-ounce 3.5cm-thick beef fillet steak or 2cm-thick sirloin steak

Add 40ml red wine

Add 150ml beef stock

Add 0.166 ounce tomato purée

Add 0.166 ounce cornflour, dissolved in 0.5 ounce water

Instructions:

The oven heats up to 430°F.

Place the potatoes in a boiling water saucepan, bring it back to the boil and cook for 4–5 minutes, then drain. Put 0.166 ounce of oil in a roasting tin and fry half an hour in a hot oven. Turn the potatoes after every 10 minutes to ensure that they cook evenly. Remove from oven when cooked, sprinkle with the chopped parsley and mix well.

Fry the onion 5–7 minutes over medium heat in 1 teaspoon of oil until soft and beautifully caramelized. Keep dry. Steam the kale, then steam for 2–3 minutes. In 1⁄2 teaspoon of oil, fry the garlic gently for 1 minute, until soft but not colored. Add the kale and fry, until tender, for another 1–2 minutes. Keep dry.

Heat a frying pan, which is ovenproof over high heat until it smokes. Cover the meat in 1⁄2 teaspoon of the oil and fry over medium-high heat in the hot pan, depending on how you like your meat cooked. If you want your meat medium, it would be easier to sear the meat and then move the pan to a 430°F oven and finish the cooking according to the prescribed times.

Remove the meat from the saucepan and put aside for rest. Add the wine to the hot saucepan to produce any meat residue—bubble to halve the liquor, to syrupy, and with a strong flavor.

Transfer the stock and tomato purée to the steak pan and bring to the boiling point, then add the cornflour paste to thicken your sauce, add it a little at a time until the texture you want has been achieved. Attach some of the remaining steak juices and eat with the roasted potatoes, spinach, onion rings, and red wine sauce.

Thoroughly mix everything together and cook over a gentle heat for 20 minutes with the lid on. When the dhal starts sticking, mix regularly, and apply a little more water.

add the kale After 20 minutes, stir thoroughly and replace the lid and cook for another 5 minutes (1-2 minutes if spinach is used instead!)

24) Kale, edamame and tofu curry

Ingredients:

0.5 ounce rapeseed oil

Add one large onion, chopped

Add four cloves garlic, peeled and grated

Add one large thumb (7cm) fresh ginger, peeled and grated

Add one red chili, deseeded and thinly sliced

Add 0.083 ounce ground turmeric

1/4 tsp cayenne pepper

0.166 ounce paprika

0.083 ounce ground cumin

0.166 ounce salt

8.8 ounce dried red lentils

1 liter boiling water

1.76 ounce frozen soyaedamame beans

7.05 ounce firm tofu, chopped into cubes

Two tomatoes, roughly chopped

Juice of 1 lime

7.05 ounce kale leaves stalk removed and torn

Instructions:

Put the oil over low-medium heat in a heavy-bottomed oven. Add the onion and cook for at least 5 minutes before inserting the garlic, ginger, and Chilli, then simmer for another 2 minutes. Add the turmeric, cayenne, cumin, paprika, and salt. Remove and mix again, before introducing the red lentils.

Pour in the boiling water and cook for 10 minutes until the curry has a thick 'porridge' consistency, then reduce the heat and cook for another 20-30 minutes.

Remove the soya beans, Tofu, and tomatoes and continue cooking for another 5 minutes. Add the juice of lime and kale leaves, then simmer until the kale is soft.

Place the buckwheat in a medium saucepan around 15 minutes until the curry is ready, and add a lot of boiling water. Bring the water back to the boiling point and cook for 10 minutes (or somewhat longer if you want softer buckwheat. Empty the buckwheat in a sieve and serve with the dhal.

25) Salmon Sirt Super Salad-Sirt food

Ingredients:

1.76 ounce rocket

Add 1.76 ounce chicory leaves

Add 3.52 ounce smoked salmon slices (you can also use lentils, cooked chicken breast or tinned tuna)

Add 80g avocado, peeled, stoned and sliced

Add 1.41 ounce celery, sliced

Add 0.70 ounce red onion, sliced

Add 0.52 ounce walnuts, chopped

Add 0.5 ounce capers

Add one large Medjool date, pitted and chopped

0.5 ounce extra-virgin olive oil

Juice ¼ lemon

0.35 ounce parsley, chopped

0.35 ounce lovage or celery leaves, chopped

Instructions:

Arrange the leaves of the salad on a large pan. Mix all the remaining ingredients and pour over the berries.

3.4 Recipes for Dinner

26) Turkey Skinny Satay Skewers

Ingredients:

Two teaspoons minced garlic

0.5 ounce crunchy peanut butter (adjust to your tastes)

1 ounce brown sugar, packed

Salt to season

8 ounce light coconut milk

0.166 ounce turmeric

1.5 ounce powdered peanut butter

21.16 ounce | one 1/2lbs turkey breast fillets, cubed

Extra water if needed

Fresh coriander leaves

12 wooden skewers

Coconut oil spray

Instructions:

30 Minutes for soaking skewers. Section turkey string onto skewers, then put back.

In a separate big, shallow dish, combine all the ingredients together and whisk until mixed. Attach skewers and marinade to a deeper taste for around an hour OR overnight.

Drain the turkey skewers while they are ready to cook, reserving the marinade. Spray the oil spray on a non-stick pan/skillet and fry over medium heat in two lots (I did 6 per batch) until the underside is browned. Move it to the other side and cook for another 4-5 minutes or until the turkey has cooked over. Alternatively, bake in a preheated oven at medium-high heat under the grill/broil settings until cooked, turning once after about 10 minutes.

Switch the reserved marinade to a small pot or saucepan and over high heat carry to a boil. Reduce heat to normal, and simmer for 5 minutes while stirring or until the sauce is fragrant and thick. (Add extra water per cubicle only if the sauce is too thick

Serve skewers with leaves of coriander, steamed rice or vegetables, and sprinkle with satay sauce.

27) Chilli with meat

Ingredients:

0.5 ounce oil

0.16 ounce heaped hot chili powder (or 1 level tbsp if you only have mild)

0.166 ounce paprika

One large onion

One red pepper

2 garlic cloves

0.166 ounce ground cumin

17.63 ounce lean minced beef

One beef stock cube

Take 0.166 ounce sugar (or add a thumbnail-sized piece of dark chocolate along with the beans instead)

1 ounce tomato purée

14.46 ounce can red kidney beans

14 ounce can chopped tomatoes

½ tsp dried marjoram

Plain boiled long grain rice, to serve

Soured cream, to serve

Instructions:

Get your vegetables ready. Chop into tiny dice one big onion, around 5 mm long. Cut the onion from root to tip in half, peel it and slice it lengthwise into thick matchsticks every half, not cutting it all the way to the root end, so they're still held together. Round into tidy dice over the match sticks.

Break one red pepper in half lengthwise, cut base, wash off the seeds, then chop. Peel and finely chop two cloves of garlic.

Kick-off cooking. Place your pan over medium heat onto the hob. Apply 0.5 ounce of oil and keep on for 1-2 minutes before heated (on an electric hob a little longer).

Cook for 5 minutes after placing onion, stirring fairly often, or until the onion is soft, squidgy, and slightly translucent.

Tip the garlic, red pepper, one heaped tsp of hot chili powder or 0.5 ounce of soft chili powder, 0.166 ounce of paprika, and 0.166 ounce of cumin ground.

Offer it a quick swirl, then leave for another 5 minutes to cook, stirring periodically.

Brown 500 g lean beef. Turn the heat up a little, add the meat to the saucepan and break it with your spatula or spoon. When you add the slimming, the mix should sizzle a little bit.

For 5 minutes, Keep stirring and prodding for at least 5

minutes, until all thinness is in uniform, thin lumps and no pink bits are left. Making sure you hold fire high enough to cook the meat and turn orange rather than just stewing.

Make some sauce. Crumble one cube of the beef reserve into 300ml of hot water. Pour it in the slimming mixture into the oven.

Add chopped tomatoes to a 14 ounce can. Cover with 1/2 tsp of dried marjoram, 0.166 ounce of sugar, and give a strong salt and pepper shake. Sprinkle with some 1 ounce of tomato purée and mix well the sauce.

Simmer softly around it. Bring the whole thing to the boil, stir well, and put a lid on the saucepan. Turn heat down and leave for 20 minutes.

Occasionally check on the pan to stir it and make sure that the sauce does not stick to the pan or dry out. If it sticks, add a few tablespoons of water and ensure that the heat is very small enough. The saucy, thin mixture should look thick, moist, and juicy after gently simmering.

Drain and rinse in a sieve a 410 g can of red kidney beans, then mix them into the chili pot. Carry to the boil again, and steam softly for another 10 minutes without the cap, adding some more water if it seems too cold.

Taste a bit of the season and Chilli. Possibly, it would require far more seasoning than you thought.

Now lift the lid, turn the heat down, and leave your Chilli to stand before serving for 10 minutes.

Serve long grain rice with soured milk and simple boiled rice.

28) Thai Red Curry

Ingredients:

Pinch of salt, more to taste

Add 0.5 ounce finely grated fresh ginger (about a 1-inch nub of ginger)

Add two cloves garlic, pressed or minced

One ¼ cups brown jasmine rice or long-grain brown rice, rinsed

0.5 ounce coconut oil or olive oil

One small white onion, chopped (about 8 ounce)

One red bell pepper, sliced into thin 2-inch long strips

One yellow, orange or green bell pepper, sliced into thin 2-inch long strips

½ cup of water

Take 1 ½ cups packed thinly sliced kale (tough ribs removed first), preferably the Tuscan/lacinato/dinosaur variety

Add 1 ½ teaspoon coconut sugar or turbinado (raw) sugar or brown sugar

0.5 ounce tamari or soy sauce

Two teaspoons rice vinegar or fresh lime juice

Three carrots, peeled and sliced on the diagonal into ¼-inch thick rounds (about 8 ounce)

1 ounce Thai red curry paste

One can (14 ounces) regular coconut milk

Garnishes: a handful of chopped fresh basil or cilantro, optional red pepper flakes, optional sriracha or chili garlic sauce

Instructions:

To cook rice, Boil a large pot of water. Add the rinsed rice and proceed to boil for 30 minutes to prevent overload, decreasing heat as required. Remove the rice from fire, drain and place the rice back in the bowl. Let the rice rest until you're ready to serve for 10 minutes or longer. Just before eating, sauté the rice with salt and fluff it with a fork to try.

To render the curry, fire up a broad skillet over medium heat with deep sides. When it's dry, then add the oil. Attach the onion and a sprinkle of salt and fry, stirring regularly for around 5 minutes until the onion has softened. Add the ginger and garlic and simmer for around 30 seconds, while constantly stirring, until fragrant.

Add chilies and carrots to the whistle. Cook, stirring regularly until the bell peppers are fork-tender, 3 to 5 more minutes. Then, apply the curry paste and cook for 2 minutes, stirring frequently.

Add milk, tea, kale, and sugar to the coconut and stir to combine. Carry the mixture over medium heat to a simmer. Reduce heat as necessary to keep a gentle simmer and cook until the peppers, carrots, and kale have softened to your liking, occasionally stirring for about 5 to 10 minutes.

Remove the pot from heat and add tamari and rice vinegar to season. Add salt (for optimal flavor, I added 1/4 teaspoon) to taste. If the curry needs a bit more punch, add 0.083 ounce more tamari, or add 1/2 teaspoon more rice vinegar for more acidity. Divide rice and curry into two bowls and garnish, if you like, with chopped cilantro and a sprinkling of red pepper flakes. Serve with sriracha sauce on the floor, whether you enjoy spicy curries.

If you want to add Tofu, bake it first and add it in phase 4 with coconut milk. If you add raw Tofu, the liquid will soak up too much, and baking it will improve the texture considerably, anyway.

29) Miso-marinated baked cod

Ingredients:

Add 3 1⁄2 teaspoons (0.70 ounce) miso

Add 0.5 ounce mirin

Add0.5 ounce extra virgin olive oil

Add1 x 7-ounce (7.05 ounce) skinless cod fillet

Add 1⁄8 cup (0.70 ounce) red onion, sliced

Add 3⁄8 cup (1.41 ounce) celery, sliced

Add two garlic cloves, finely chopped

Add 1 Thai chili, finely chopped

Add 0.166 ounce finely chopped fresh ginger

Add 3⁄8 cup (2.11 ounce) green beans

Add 3⁄4 cup (1.76 ounce) kale, roughly chopped

Add 0.166 ounce sesame seeds

Add 1 ounce(0.17 ounce) parsley, roughly chopped

Add 0.5 ounce tamari (or soy sauce, if not avoiding gluten)

Add 1⁄4 cup (1.41 ounce) buckwheat

0.166 ounce ground turmeric

Instructions:

Mix the 0.166 ounce of oil with the miso and mirin.

Rub the cod all over, and leave for 30 minutes to marinate. Heat the oven to 425°F.

Bake the cod for about 10 minutes.

Meanwhile, bring the remaining oil to a large frying pan or wok. Stir-fry the onion for a few minutes, then incorporate the celery, garlic, chili, ginger, green beans, and kale. Toss and fry until the kale is cooked clean and soft. To help the cooking process, you might need to add a little water to the pan.

Cook the buckwheat along with the turmeric according to the packet directions.

To the stir-fry, add the sesame seeds, parsley, and tamari and serve with buckwheat and fish.

30) Aromatic chicken breast with kale

Ingredients:

Add 1⁄4 pound (4.23 ounce) skinless, boneless chicken breast

Add two teaspoons ground turmeric

juice of 1⁄4 lemon

Add 0.5 ounce extra virgin olive oil

Add 3⁄4 cup (1.76 ounce) kale, chopped

Add 1⁄8 cup (0.70 ounce) red onion, sliced

0.166 ounce chopped fresh ginger

1⁄3 cup (1.76 ounce) buckwheat

For the sauce:

Take one medium tomato (130g)

Add 1 Thai chili, finely chopped

Add 0.5 ounce capers, finely chopped

Add 1 ounce(0.17 ounce) parsley, finely chopped

Add the juice of 1/4 lemon

Instructions:

Remove the eye from the tomato and finely chop it to make the salsa, taking great care to maintain the maximum amount of fluid. Pair chili, capers, lemon juice with the mixture. You could put it all in a mixer, but the final result is a little different.

To 425°F, heat the oven. In 1 teaspoon of turmeric, marinate the chicken breast with lemon juice and a little butter. Leave for five to ten minutes.

Take the marinated chicken and heat until hot in the ovenproof pan for about 1-10 minutes on each side. Then, transform it into an oven (place it on a bakery, if the pot is ovenproof) and cook until it is golden pale for about 8 to 10 minutes. Recover and leave to rest 5 minutes prior to serving from the oven.

In the meantime, cook the kale for 5 minutes in a steamer. Fry in some oil the red onions and ginger, then add the cooked pulp and fry for a further minute until soft but not browned.

Cook buckwheat with the remaining turmeric teaspoon according to the package instructions. Serve chicken, herbs, and salsa together.

31) Asian shrimp stir-fry with buckwheat noodles

Ingredients:

Take 1/3 pound (5.29 ounce) shelled raw jumbo shrimp, deveined

Add two teaspoons tamari (you can use soy sauce if you are not avoiding gluten)

Two teaspoons extra virgin olive oil

3 ounces (2.64 ounce) soba (buckwheat noodles)

Two garlic cloves, finely chopped

Add 1 Thai chili, finely chopped

Add 0.166 ounce finely chopped fresh ginger

Take 1/8 cup (0.70 ounce) red onions, sliced

Add 1/2 cup (45g) celery including leaves, trimmed and sliced, with leaves set aside

1/2 cup (2.64 ounce) green beans, chopped

3/4 cup (1.76 ounce) kale, roughly chopped

1/2 cup (3.38 ounce) chicken stock

Instructions:

Heat a frying pan by placing over high heat, then cook the shrimp for 2 to 3 minutes in 0.5 ounce tamari and 0.166 ounce oil.

Shift to a plate the shrimp. Wipe out the pan with a towel of ink because you can again use it.

Cook the noodles 5-8 minutes, or according to product directions, in boiling water. Remove and reserve.

Meanwhile, fry on medium-high heat for 3 minutes in the remaining tamari, chile, ginger, red onion, celery (but not the leaves), green beans, and kale. Place the stock and let it boil until the vegetables are cooked but still crunchy. Cook for a minute or two, then simmer.

Add the shrimp, noodles, and celery to the pot, bring them back to a boil, and then remove them from the heat.

32) Turmeric chicken & kale salad

Ingredients

To make chicken

Add1 teaspoon ghee or 0.5 ounce coconut oil

Add ½ medium brown onion, diced

Take 250-300 g / 9 oz. chicken mince or diced up chicken thighs

Add one large garlic clove, finely diced

Add 0.166 ounce turmeric powder

Add 1teaspoon lime zest

Add the juice of ½ lime

Add ½ teaspoon salt + pepper

For the salad

Add six broccolini stalks or 2 cups of broccoli florets

Add 1 ounce pumpkin seeds (pepitas)

Add three large kale leaves, stems removed and chopped

Add ½ avocado, sliced

Add a handful of fresh coriander leaves, chopped

Add a handful of fresh parsley leaves, chopped

For the dressing

Add 1.5 ounce lime juice

Add one small garlic clove, finely diced or grated

Add 1.5 ounce extra-virgin olive oil

Add 0.166 ounce raw honey

Add ½ teaspoon wholegrain or Dijon mustard

Add ½ teaspoon sea salt and pepper

Instructions:

Take a small frying pan, heat the ghee or coconut oil over medium to high heat. Insert the onion and sauté for 4-5 minutes on medium heat, until golden. Add the minced chicken and garlic and stir over medium-high heat for 2-3 minutes, breaking it apart.

Add the lime zest, turmeric, lime juice, salt, and pepper and cook for a further 3-4 minutes, stirring frequently. Set aside the fried slush.

Use a pan filled with water to boil while the chicken cooks. Stir in the broccolini and cook 2 minutes. Rinse under cold water and cut into three to four pieces each.

Put the pumpkin seeds from the chicken into the frying pan and toast for 2 minutes over medium heat, stirring periodically to avoid burning—season to a touch of water. Deposit back. Raw pumpkin seeds should also be good for use.

In a salad bowl, put the chopped kale, and pour over the dressing. Toss the kale with the sauce, then rub it with your palms. This should loosen the kale, kind of like what citrus juice does to carpaccio fish or beef – it 'cooks' it a little bit.

The fried rice, broccolini, new basil, pumpkin seeds, and slices of avocado are eventually tossed.

33) Buckwheat noodles with chicken kale & miso dressing

Ingredients:

For the noodles

Take 2-3 handfuls of kale leaves (removed from the stem and roughly cut)

Add 5.29 ounce / 5 oz buckwheat noodles (100% buckwheat, no wheat)

Add 3-4 shiitake mushrooms, sliced

Add 0.166 ounce coconut oil or ghee

Add one brown onion, finely diced

Add one medium free-range chicken breast, sliced or diced

Add one long red chili, thinly sliced (seeds in or out depending on how hot you like it)

Add two large garlic cloves, finely diced

Add 2-3 tablespoons Tamari sauce (gluten-free soy sauce)

For the miso dressing

Add 1½ tablespoon fresh organic miso

Add 0.5 ounce Tamari sauce

Add 0.5 ounce extra-virgin olive oil

Add0.5 ounce lemon or lime juice

Add 0.166 ounce sesame oil (optional)

Instructions:

To boil water, bring a medium saucepan. Add the kale and cook for at least 1 minute. Remove and put aside, then carry the water back to the boil. Attach the soba noodles and cook (usually around 5 minutes) according to package directions. Set aside and rinse under cold water.

Meanwhile, in a little ghee or coconut oil (about a teaspoon), pan fry the shiitake mushrooms for 2-3 minutes, until well browned on either side. Sprinkle with sea salt and set aside.

Heat more coconut oil or ghee in the same frying pan over medium to high heat. Stir in onion and Chilli for 2-3 minutes, then add pieces of chicken. Cook over medium heat for 5 minutes, stirring a few times, then add the garlic, tamari sauce, and some splash of water. Cook for another 2-3 minutes, often stirring until chicken is cooked completely.

At last, add the kale and soba noodles and warm up by stirring through the chicken.

At the end of the cooking, mix the miso dressing and drizzle over the noodles to keep all the beneficial probiotics alive and active in the miso.

34) Asian king prawn stir-fry with buckwheat noodles

Ingredients:

Take 5.29 ounce shelled raw king prawns, deveined

Add 2 tsp tamari (you can use soy sauce if you are not avoiding gluten)

2 tsp extra virgin olive oil

2.64 ounce soba (buckwheat noodles)

One garlic clove, finely chopped

One bird's eye chili, finely chopped

0.166 ounce finely chopped fresh ginger

0.70 ounce red onions, sliced

1.41 ounce celery, trimmed and sliced

2.64 ounce green beans, chopped

1.76 ounce kale, roughly chopped

3.38 ounce chicken stock

0.17 ounce lovage or celery leaves

Instructions:

Heat a frying pan over a high temperature, then cook the prawns for 2-3 minutes in 1 teaspoon tamari and 0.166 ounce oil. Put the prawns onto a plate. Wipe the pan out with paper from the kitchen, as you will be using it again.

Cook the noodles 5-8 minutes in boiling water, or as indicated on the package. Drain and pack away.

Meanwhile, over a medium-high fire, fry the garlic, Chilli and ginger, red onion, celery, beans, and kale in the remaining oil for 4-5 minutes. Add the stock and bring to the boiling point, then cook for one or two minutes until the vegetables are cooked but crunchy.

Transfer the prawns, noodles, and leaves of lovage/celery to the oven put back to the simmer, then reduce the heat and drink.

35) Baked salmon salad with creamy mint dressing

Ingredients:

One salmon fillet (130g)

1.41 ounce mixed salad leaves

1.41 ounce young spinach leaves

Two radishes, trimmed and thinly sliced

5cm piece (1.76 ounce) cucumber, cut into chunks

Two spring onions, trimmed and sliced

One small handful (0.35 ounce) parsley, roughly chopped

For the dressing:

0.166 ounce low-fat mayonnaise

0.5 ounce natural yogurt

0.5 ounce rice vinegar

Two leaves mint, finely chopped

Salt and freshly ground black pepper

Instructions:

Oven preheated to 390°F.

Transform salmon to a baking tray and bake for 16–18 minutes until you have just cooked. Delete and put aside from the oven. The salmon in the salad is equally nice and hot or cold. If your salmon has skin, just cook the skin side down and remove the salmon from the skin after cooking, using a slice of fish. When cooked, it will slip away quickly.

Put the mayonnaise, mustard, rice wine vinegar, mint leaves, and salt and pepper together in a small bowl and leave to stand for at least 5 minutes to make

Aromas to grow.

Place on a serving plate the lettuce leaves and spinach, then finish with the radishes, the cucumber, the spring onions, and the parsley. Flake the cooked salmon over the salad and sprinkle over the dressing.

36) Fragrant Asian Hotpot-Sirtfood recipe

Ingredients:

Add 0.166 ounce tomato purée

Add 1-star anise, crushed (or 1/4 tsp ground anise)

Small handful (0.35 ounce) parsley, stalks finely chopped

Small handful (1Og) coriander, stalks finely chopped

Juice of 1/2 lime

500ml chicken stock, fresh or made with one cube

Add 1/2 carrot, peeled and cut into matchsticks

Take 1.76 ounce broccoli, cut into small florets

Add 1.76 ounce beansprouts

Add 1OOg raw tiger prawns

Add 1OOg firm tofu, chopped

Add 1.76 ounce rice noodles, cooked according to packet instructions

Add 1.76 ounce cooked water chestnuts, drained

Add 0.70 ounce sushi ginger, chopped

Add 0.5 ounce good-quality miso paste

Instructions:

In a wide saucepan, put the tomato purée, star anise, parsley stalks, coriander stalks, lime juice, and chicken.

Stir in the cabbage, broccoli, prawns, Tofu, pasta, and water chestnuts and simmer gently before the prawns are finished. Remove from stove and mix in the ginger sushi and the paste miso.

Serve mixed with the leaves of the parsley and coriander.

37) Lamb, butternut squash and date Tagine-Sirtfood recipe

Ingredients:

Add 1 ounce olive oil

Add one red onion, sliced

Add 2cm ginger, grated

Three garlic cloves, grated or crushed

0.166 ounce chili flakes (or to taste)

2 teaspoons cumin seeds

One cinnamon stick

Two teaspoons ground turmeric

Take 800g lamb neck fillet, cut into 2cm chunks

Add ½ teaspoon salt

Add 3.52 ounce Medjool dates, pitted and chopped

Add 14 ounce tin chopped tomatoes, plus half a can of water

Add 17.63 ounce butternut squash, chopped into 1cm cubes

Add 14 ounce tin chickpeas, drained

1 ounce fresh coriander (plus extra for garnish)

Buckwheat, couscous, flatbreads or rice to serve

Instructions:

Preheat the oven to 280°F.

Drizzle around two teaspoons of olive oil in a large ovenproof saucepan. Take the sliced onion and cook on a gentle heat until the onions are softened but not brown, with the lid on for about 5 minutes.

Add Chilli, cumin, cinnamon, and turmeric to the grated garlic and ginger. Mix well, and cook the lid off for one more minute. If it gets too dry, add a splash of water.

Next, introduce pieces of lamb. In the onions and spices, mix well to cover the meat and then apply butter, diced dates, and tomatoes, plus around half a can of water (3.38-6.76 ounce).

Carry the tagine to the simmer, then place the cover on and position it for 1 hour and 15 minutes in your preheated oven.

Add the sliced butternut squash and drained chickpeas thirty minutes until the end of the cooking period. Stir all together, put the lid back on and go back to the oven for the final 30 minutes of cooking.

Remove from the oven when the tagine is prepared, and mix through the chopped coriander. Serve with couscous, buckwheat, flatbreads, or basmati rice.

38) Prawn Arrabbiata-Sirtfood recipe

Ingredients:

Take 4.40-5.29 ounce Raw or cooked prawns (Ideally king prawns)

Take 65 g Buckwheat pasta

0.5 ounce Extra virgin olive oil

For arrabbiata sauce

1.4 ounce Red onion, finely chopped

1 Garlic clove, finely chopped

3.05 ounce Celery, finely chopped

1 Bird's eye chili, finely chopped

0.166 ounce Dried mixed herbs

0.166 ounce Extra virgin olive oil

1 ounce White wine (optional)

14 ounce Tinned chopped tomatoes

0.5 ounce Chopped parsley

Instructions:

1. Fry the onion, garlic, celery, and chili over medium-low heat and dried herbs in the oil for 1-2 minutes. Turn down the heat to normal, then add the wine and cook for a minute. Add the tomatoes and let the sauce cook over medium-low heat for 20-30 minutes until it has a good, rich consistency. Add some water if sauce is too thick.

While the sauce is heating, bring a pan of water to the boil and cook the pasta as instructed by the packet. Drain, toss with the olive oil when cooked to your liking, and keep in the pan until needed.

Add the raw prawns to the sauce and cook for another 3-4 minutes until they have turned pink and opaque, then add the parsley and serve. If you use cooked prawns, add the parsley, bring the sauce to the boil and serve.

Add the sauce in the cooked pasta and mix well but gently and serve.

3.5 Assorted Recipes

Salads

39) Vegan Kale Salad with Cranberries

Ingredients:

¼ cup dried cranberries

One dash salt optional

¼ cup pine nuts or other chopped nuts optional

6 cups of shredded Kale

1/3 cup Maple Vinaigrette Dressing

Instructions:

Clean the Kale.

Rip it into tiny bits that remove the rough core.

Place the Maple Vinaigrette Dressing in a wide bowl and drizzle over.

Sprinkle with a bit of salt

Massage the dressing onto the kale with your palms until it becomes bright green and shiny.

If needed, scatter with dried cranberries, and finish with nuts.

40) Coronation chicken salad

Ingredients:

Add 75 g Natural yogurt

Juice of 1/4 of a lemon

0.166 ounce Coriander, chopped

0.166 ounce ground turmeric

0.083 ounce Mild curry powder

Take 3.52 ounce Cooked chicken breast, cut into bite-sized pieces

6 Walnut halves, finely chopped

1 Medjool date, finely chopped

0.70 ounce Red onion, diced

1 Bird's eye chili

1.4 ounce Rocket, to serve

Instructions:

Mix the lemon juice, yogurt, coriander, and spices together in a bowl. Serve on a bed of rocket by adding all the other ingredients.

41) Buckwheat pasta sald

Ingredients:

Take 1.76 ounce buckwheat pasta(cooked according to the packet instructions)

large handful of rocket

A small handful of basil leaves

Eight cherry tomatoes halved

1/2 avocado, diced

Ten olives

0.5 ounce extra virgin olive oil

0.70 ounce pine nuts

Instructions:

Except for pine nuts, add all the ingredients and arrange in a bowl, then scatter the pine nuts over the top.

42) Greek salad skewers

Ingredients:

Take two wooden skewers, soaked in water for 30 minutes before use

Add eight large black olives

Add eight cherry tomatoes

Add one yellow pepper, cut into eight squares

Add ½ red onion, cut in half and separated into eight pieces

Add 3.52 ounce (about 10cm) cucumber, cut into four slices and halved

3.52 ounce feta, cut into eight cubes

For the dressing:

Add 0.5 ounce extra virgin olive oil

Add the juice of ½ lemon

Add 0.166 ounce balsamic vinegar

Take ½ clove garlic, peeled and crushed

Add Few leaves of basil, finely chopped (or ½ tsp dried mixed herbs to replace basil and oregano)

Few leaves oregano, finely chopped

you can doa seasoning of salt and freshly ground black pepper

Instructions:

Thread each skewer in the order with salad ingredients: olive, tomato, yellow pepper, red onion, cucumber, feta, tomato, olive, yellow pepper, red ointment, cucumber, feta.

Place all the ingredients of the dressing in a small bowl and mix well together. Pour over the skewers.

43) Sesame chicken salad

Ingredients:

Take 0.5 ounce sesame seeds

Add one cucumber, peeled, halved lengthways, deseeded with a teaspoon and sliced

3.52 ounce baby kale, roughly chopped

2.11 ounce pak choi, very finely shredded

½ red onion, very finely sliced

Large handful (0.70 ounce) parsley, chopped

5.29 ounce cooked chicken, shredded

For the dressing:

0.5 ounce extra virgin olive oil

0.166 ounce sesame oil

Juice of 1 lime

0.166 ounce clear honey

2 tsp soy sauce

Instructions:

Toast the sesame seeds for 2 minutes until lightly browned and fragrant. Pass to cool board.

Blend the olive oil, sesame oil, lime juice, honey, and soy sauce together in a small bowl to create a dressing.

Put the cucumber, kale, Choi pak, red onion, and parsley in a wide bowl and combine gently. Rub over the coating, then again blend.

Spread the salad with the grilled chicken between two plates on top. Just before eating, scatter over the sesame seeds.

44) Chicory and Nut Salad

Ingredients:

0.083 ounce Dijon mustard

Salt and freshly ground black pepper

8 ounce chicory, or other leafy green

2 ounce shaved Parmesan

4 ounce coarsely chopped walnuts

0.5 ounce sherry vinegar

1.5 ounce walnut oil

Instructions:

Add the nuts in a dry skillet over medium-high heat until they are fragrant, around 2 minutes. Put aside to cool down.

Whisk the vinegar, sugar, mustard, salt, and pepper together in a tiny cup to match.

Place the chicory in a wide bowl with the covering. Put

walnuts on the serving plates for topping as well as shaved Parmesan.

Drinks and Juices

45) The Sirt food Juice

Ingredients:

Two large handfuls (2.64 ounce) kale

A very small handful (0.17 ounce) flat-leaf parsley

A large handful (1.05 ounce) rocket

Take A very small handful (0.17 ounce) lovage leaves (optional)

Add 2–3 large stalks (5.29 ounce) green celery, including its leaves

½ medium green apple

½ level tsp matcha green tea

Juice of ½ lemon

Instructions:

Mix together the greens (kale, rocket, parsley, and lovage, if used), then sauté them. I have found that juicers can really differ in their efficiency when juicing leafy vegetables, and before moving on to the other ingredients, you may need to re-juice the remains. The target is to finish off the greens with about 50ml of water.

Now you can peel the lemon and also put it through the juicer, but I find simply squeezing lemon in the juice by hand convenient. You should have about 8.4 ounces of juice in total by this stage, maybe a little bit more. It's only when the juice is made and ready to serve that you add the green tea matcha.

In a glass, pour a small amount of juice, then add the matcha, and stir vigorously with a fork or teaspoon. For the first two drinks of the day, we only use matcha because it contains small amounts of caffeine (similar to a normal teacup). Once the matcha is absorbed, add the remainder of the drink, it can hold them alive for people not used to it.

Give it a stirring finish, and then your juice is ready to drink. Free to top up with plain water, as you like.

46) Grape and melon juice-Sirtfood recipe

Ingredients:

Take ½ cucumber, peeled if preferred, halved, seeds removed and roughly chopped

Add 1.05 ounce young spinach leaves, stalks removed

Add 3.52 ounce red seedless grapes

Add 3.52 ounce cantaloupe melon, peeled, deseeded and cut into chunks

Instructions:

Mix thoroughly in a juicer or blender until smooth.

47) Kale and blackcurrant smoothie

Ingredients:

2 tsp honey

8 ounce freshly made green tea

Ten baby kale leaves stalk removed

One ripe banana

1.4 ounce blackcurrants, washed and stalks removed

Six ice cubes

Instructions:

Add honey into green tea and mix until dissolved. Add ingredients in a blender and mix until smooth. Serve immediately.

48) Green Tea Smoothie

This super-healthy smoothie contains matcha powder, which is a type of Japanese green tea. It can be found in Asian tea shops.

Ingredients:

Two ripe bananas

250 ml of milk

Add 2 tsp matcha green tea powder

Add 1/2 tsp vanilla bean paste (not extract) or a small scrape of the seeds from a vanilla pod

Six ice cubes

2 tsp honey

Instructions:

Just mix all the ingredients together in a blender and serve in two glasses.

49) Ginger Turmeric Lemonade

New ginger turmeric lemonade recipe rendered whole foods: raw ginger and turmeric root and a touch of black peppercorns to improve curcumin absorption and enhance the buds of the palate.

Ingredients:

Four lemons

Take 7 cups of filtered water

Add 1.5-inch turmeric root (or 2 tsp turmeric powder)

Add 1-inch ginger root (or more to taste)

12 peppercorns

1/4 cup coconut nectar or six dates

Instructions:

Split the lemons slice off with a small knife. Remove the seeds, then add the lemons to a strong food processor or blender.

Peel the root of the turmeric and ginger and transfer them together with the peppercorns and sweetener or according to preference to the blender.

Grinding until smooth. You can taste it and adjust sweetness according to flavor.

Serve over ice, chilled.

Sweets

50) Chocolate Nut truffles

Ingredients:

Take 0.5 ounce Frangelico or 0.166 ounce vanilla extract

1.76 ounce hazelnut, roughly chopped

175ml double cream

7.05 ounce bar dark chocolate, finely chopped

different colored sprinkles and edible glitters

Instructions:

Heat milk until it reaches a boiling point in a tiny saucepan. Remove from the flame and dump the minced chocolate over it. Stir the mixture gently until dry, then add the extract of alcohol or coffee, and the hazelnuts. Place in a refrigerator by covering for 30 minutes, or until dense but not solid.

Scoop out the mixture's teaspoons and form with your hands into little spheres. Place each of your sprinkles or glitters on different plaques or containers. Roll each truffle to cover in the sprinkles or shimmer, then chill again to firm up. Will keep it chilled for one week, or freeze without decoration for up to 1 month.

51) Chocolate Balls

Ingredients:

14 ounce can condensed milk

4 ounce desiccated coconut

7.05 ounce Arrowroot biscuits crushed

1.5 ounce cacao powder

Instructions:

Mix together the broken biscuit, chocolate, and condensed milk to create a sticky consistency.

Using a generous mixture tablespoon, shape into balls and wrap in coconut.

Chill it before you drink.

52) Crème Brulee

Ingredients:

8 ounce vanilla sugar, divided

Six large egg yolks

2 quarts hot water

1-quart heavy cream

One vanilla bean split and scraped

Instructions:

Preheat the oven to 325°F.

Place the milk, vanilla bean and pulp in a medium-high heat saucepan and bring to a boil. Remove from the heat, cover, and allow for 15 minutes of sitting. Remove the vanilla bean and set aside for further use.

Whisk 4 ounce sugar and the egg yolks together in a medium bowl until well mixed until it only begins to lighten in color. Apply the milk, constantly mixing, a little at a time. Pour the liquid into six ramekins (7 to 8-ounce) Place the ramekins in a large cake saucepan or roast pan. Pour enough hot water into the saucepan to halfway up the sides of the ramekins. Bake for about 40 to 45 minutes until the creme Brulee is set but still trembling in the center.

Extract the ramekins from the roasting pan and refrigerate for a total of two hours at least and up to three days. Remove the creme Brulee from the fridge for at least 30 minutes until the sugar has browned on top. Uniformly Divide the remaining 4 ounceof vanilla sugar across the six plates and evenly scatter across the rim. Melt the sugar using a flame, then shape a crispy layer. Enable the creme Brulee to sit for 5 minutes or more before serving.

52) Sirt food bites (makes 15-20 bites)

Ingredients:

1.05 ounce dark chocolate, broken into pieces; or cocoa nibs

8.8 ounce Medjool dates pitted

4.23 ounce walnuts

0.5 ounce cocoa powder

Take The scraped seeds of 1 vanilla pod or 0.166 ounce vanilla extract

Add 0.5-1 ounce water

0.5 ounce ground turmeric

0.5 ounce extra virgin olive oil

Instructions:

Add walnuts and chocolate in a blender and process them until the powder is perfect.

Add all the other ingredients except water and mix until

a ball forms the mixture. On the basis of the consistency of the mixture, you may or may not have to add the water; you don't want it to be too sticky.

Shape the mixture into bite-sized balls with your hands, then refrigerate for at least 1 hour in an airtight jar before consuming them. In some more cocoa or desiccated coconut, you could roll some of the balls to achieve a different finish if you like. They will keep it in your fridge for up to 1 week.

53) Chocolate cupcakes with matcha icing

Ingredients:

5.3-ounce self-rising flour

7.05-ounce caster sugar

2.1-ounce cocoa

0.083-ounce salt

0.083-ounce fine espresso coffee, decaf if preferred

4.05-ounce milk

0.083-ounce vanilla extract

1.7-ounce vegetable oil

One egg

4.05 ounce boiling water

For the icing:

1.7-ounces butter, at room temperature

1.7-ounce icing sugar

0.5-ounce matcha green tea powder

0.083-ounce vanilla bean paste

1.7-ounces soft cream cheese

Instructions:

Preheat the fan for the oven to 320°F/350°F. Form a paper or silicone cake case of a cupcake tray.

In a wide pot, place the rice, sugar, chocolate, salt, and espresso powder and thoroughly blend.

Add the dry ingredients with the sugar, vanilla extract, vegetable oil, and egg, then use an electric mixer to beat until well mixed. Pour in the boiling water gently gradually and pump at low velocity before completely mixed. Using a high-velocity beat to introduce oxygen to the batter for another minute. The batter is much more acidic than a regular cake mix. Have confidence; it'll taste amazing!

In the cake instances, scoop the batter equally. Per cake box should be no more than 3⁄4 complete. Bake for 15-18 minutes in the oven, before the mixture, bounces back when pressed. Take it out from the oven and let it cool until icing fully.

Mix butter and icing sugar together until light and dry to create the icing.

Remove the coffee and matcha powder, then mix again. Remove the cream cheese, then beat until smooth. Pip or sprinkle over the cakes.

CHAPTER 04: MAINTAINING WEIGHT AFTER SIRT FOOD DIET

4.1 Build up Your Strength

When you think of the best type of weight loss workouts, your mind may not jump to the strength training immediately, but it should. Although it's certainly true that aerobic exercises make the heart function faster and, as a consequence, help the body lose calories, strength training is what can actually offer the weight-loss goals the boost extra.

We want to make it clear before we really venture into it that weight loss as a goal is not inherently for everybody. For someone with a history of an eating disorder, particularly though you're in rehab, you can talk to a psychiatrist before following some aim of weight-loss, even initiating a new workout regimen. So even though you don't have a history of eating disordered, it's very necessary to set reasonable standards to ensure you're maintaining a safe weight loss. Results can be extremely challenging to achieve, can take a long time to obtain, and can even be very complicated to manage. Often important to remember: only half of the calculation is the workout. To lose weight, you need to create a calorie deficit (burning more calories than you consume in a day), which requires not only working out but also being aware of what you are eating, making sure you eat quality calories, and watch portion sizes. You have to sleep well, daily. The stress levels need to be lowered. You need to look after all your own bodily needs. With so many factors at stake, weight loss is, no doubt, a very special experience for any individual.

If weight reduction is your target, it's important to integrate strength training into your routine. Although strength training does not give you the immediate heart-pounding, sweat-dripping gratification of, say, Zumba, or an indoor fitness workout, developing lean muscle certainly works against your weight-loss goals in the long run.

Strength training helps build lean muscle.

"Aerobic exercise is actually the most effective way to lose weight, but it's not the best way to burn fat and increase lean mass (muscle)," says T.S. Fitness founder Noam Tamir, C.S.C.S. It's natural to lose muscle and fat while you are losing weight solely by cardio. And if strength exercise is not part of the strategy to combat this, you may potentially be slowing down your metabolism by reducing lean muscle mass rather than reviving it up (which may lead to plateaus of weight loss).

As Michaela Devries-Aboud, Ph.D., an exercise physiologist at McMaster University, states, strength training is even effective at constructing muscle than a cardio-only regimen. "When you raise weights, you overwhelm the muscle, so it tries to adjust and carry more weight. That's by raising something called myofibrillary scale (the muscle's contractile units), how the muscle adapts," she describes. Resistance training stimulates this growth, which in time results in an increase in muscle mass. "And while aerobic exercise will [stimulate this process] as well, this improvement is not as strong as with exercise in resistance."

More muscle = a higher B.M.R. (base metabolic rate).

Having a leaner muscle ensures that the body consumes

more calories at rest. Having more muscle increases the metabolic rate of your everyday base, or B.M.R. "The muscle mass is a metabolically more costly organ,"

Devries-Aboud says. "A pound of muscle's caloric requirement is higher than it is for a pound of fat because even lying around, the volume of energy required to sustain a pound of muscle a day is higher than that of a pound of fat. Having more muscle mass will result in the consumption of more calories.

"The muscle is continuously breaking down, recreated and synthesized, and all such processes need energy. So, you're stoking the fires of your metabolism by building more muscle. You're also increasing your calorie deficit by increasing your B.M.R. and burning more calories at rest, which is necessary for weight loss. (Head here for all the calculations and details you need to find out how many calories you can need in order to lose weight.)

And don't panic if you don't see huge scale results: "Go through how your clothes fit because muscle is more compact than fat," Devries-Aboud suggests. If you don't lose as much weight as you believe you want to be, you actually develop muscle while you lose fat, and that's a positive thing! (And no, you're not going to get bumpy.)

"That new muscle has a great impact on decreasing body fat," tells Holly Perkins. "The net result is you're tighter and leaner, whatever the scale says."

You will continue burning calories during a strength workout.

Even though exercise receives a lot of attention when it comes to calorie-torching exercises, by throwing in some heart-pumping components, you will also get a decent burn during a strength-training session.

There are some items that you should do to improve your burn, Perkins says: switch between exercises quicker, don't stop between sessions, push rapidly through each session, increasing your reps, and pick heavier weights (but don't go too hard, of course, that you risk injury).

Or, "apply a five-minute aerobic interval in motions with strength: get on the treadmill and jog or run for five minutes," Perkins suggests.

"Mostly because these methods increase your heart rate during a workout," she explains. "A heart rate rise implies a greater need for fuel, and a greater need for fuel indicates the body may consume more calories. Indeed, the excess after exercise oxygen intake, or E.P.O.C., can [go up and] result in more calories being consumed during the workout, as a consequence of vigorous training. Think of E.P.O.C. as a brief boost to the metabolism. "The afterburn effect is recognized like this.

Add strength training into your weight-loss plan.

You still have to burn more calories at the end of the day than you take in to lose weight, and while building muscle can help keep that up for the long term, it's still important to chip away on a daily basis with calories. "To have a challenging cardiovascular routine helps with your caloric deficit," Tamir says.

Story morals: Do both strength training and cardio training, Tamir says. The inclusion of both types of training is important in a successful weight-loss plan. Tamir usually suggests intensity exercise for 45 to 60 minutes, three or four days a week. "Physical exercise also allows you the opportunity to stay longer through your aerobic preparation," Tamir says. "The healthier you become, the less energy aerobic exercise requires to achieve."

This ensures you will improve your efficiency in cardio-based activities: "For starters, using powerful glutes to run makes you move quicker and longer, which can burn more calories. And performing workouts to reinforce the heart will help you retain bike shape that will also help you burn more calories," says Tamir.

So no reason to abandon the aerobic dance or treadmill workout — just add a few weights into the routine, too, a couple of days a week.

4.2 Self-monitor

Self-monitoring relates to the assessment and documentation of habits of feeding and exercising, accompanied by input on behaviors. The aim of self-monitoring is to improve the self-awareness of desired habits and effects, and if issues occur, it will act as an early warning mechanism and help track the progress. Several self-monitoring strategies which are widely used include:

Food diaries

Exercise logs

Regular self-weighing

Equipment such as pedometers, accelerometers, and metabolic devices

Food Logs

In weight loss systems, one of the most popular and effective forms of self-monitoring techniques is to maintain a food journal in which individuals report meals, workouts, or drinks as soon as they are ingested.

One important technique with food logs is to record what they eat or drink as consumed, or it will not give an accurate account of the intake of the day. For food logs, a good "thumb rule" is: "if you bite it, you write it down!"

The minimal weight-loss detail that should be maintained in food records is the amount, quantity, and calorie value of the eaten food or drink. This offers the opportunity to monitor and compare the number of calories eaten all day long with the number of calories spent all day long.

Many dietary details that can be reported include feeding time of day, fat content, and grams of carbohydrate. Logs of foods specific to the disease may also be kept. For example, they are focusing on carbohydrate content in patients with diabetes or insulin resistance, instead of calories.

Food Diaries

Another useful self-monitoring tool is maintaining a food diary. Food diaries differ from food logs because more detailed information is included. They are useful if you are trying to find behavioral reasons or psychological aspects of eating.

Any food diaries may contain the stress level, mood, or emotions around feeding, action or location, or other environmental or emotional reasons to eat, depending on the individual and behavioral nuances involved. The more complex or informative the input is, the greater.

Nevertheless, in today's culture, maintaining extremely accurate everyday food reports in the long term is virtually difficult for most citizens, so enforcement with comprehensive food diaries is also very small. So large areas of concern for dietary and behavioral therapy will be identified by recommending that patients maintain a comprehensive list of diet for a few days per week.

Through this link **https://bit.ly/3d6eRT5** (write it on your internet browser), you can download for free and print a practical diary, with which you can keep track of your meals and your progress for 30 days. If you like the template, you can find some diaries in Paperback format with different covers on my Amazon page.

Logging Your Food Online

In our technologically advanced world, online food logs and diaries or computer software are quick and convenient ways to keep records of food consumed. Many websites are available throughout the day for tracking food and calories, some of which are free and very user friendly.

In online databases of more than 50,000 foods, you can look up food choices and/or alternatives. Web-savvy loggers may opt to keep their journals online.

Some may also want to use such websites as a more easy way to look up food nutritional information. Any online diaries are free and include:

www.myfooddiary.com

www.sparkpeople.com

Free diet knowledge search services are open, as an example is www.calorieking.com. Such websites can also provide monitoring and suggestions for workouts, encouragement, motivational advice, and chat rooms or rooms for discussion.

Hand-held Calorie Counters

The portable calorie counting apps are another choice for those that are "on the go." Some of the devices, like CalorieSmart ® or HealthFitCounter ®, are stand-alone. Others have to communicate with Web pages. Other apps, such as the Calorie King Diet Journal, are mounted in your Palm or Pocket-PC. They allow you to download updates when nutrition facts change, but some use a lot of memory.

Regular Weighing

Weighing yourself is an important and simple behavior of self-monitoring that serves as a reminder of one's eating and activity habits. Although weighing yourself while losing weight can be difficult and sometimes discouraging, it is recommended that you weigh yourself on the same scale weekly, preferably outside the home.

It could be more effective than home scales to use the device at the nearest gym or fitness room or the doctor's office. If this is impractical, however, it's okay to use a home scale. Try to weigh yourself on the same daytime and the same weekday.

It can help you keep track of your success or help you get back on track faster by writing down your weekly weights on a table, graph, or calendar. It is necessary to remember that it is not advised to weigh oneself more often than a week because day-to-day variations are not real weight markers. Regular weight monitoring is also essential to help you keep your weight off after weight loss.

Exercise Logs

Another self-monitoring technique is keeping an exercise log or diary along the same lines as the food logs and diaries. Ideally, the number of minutes involved and the type and level of physical activity exertion should be recorded.

An important aspect of exercise logs, which is often forgotten, is the level of perceived exertion. Walking for 30 minutes can result in varying rates of calories burned and cardiovascular effects at a quick pace compared with a hard speed.

Typically, the pace you stroll to work or go shopping will typically be a simple aerobic exercise that doesn't raise heart rate significantly or change breathing. Moderate rates of physical exertion are where you have a marginally elevated pulse rate and respiration rate. Sweating, elevated heart pressure (target heart rate range), and accelerated breathing will indicate a high or intense amount of physical exertion.

Know, it's easy to perform a physical exercise at one point or intermittently during the day. Logging may be a constructive reinforcement or encouragement to add more fitness or physical activity into the daily routine.

You are walking, riding a stationary bike, or swimming at a slow pace, maybe the initial activities. Dancing, exercise videos or chair exercises are other types of exercise that can be fun. For certain days of the week, you can strive to reach for 30 minutes of exercise.

Many people try on three or four days of the week to start exercising. However, if you can practice most of all days of the week, even if it's only 10 or 15 minutes long, it will become more of a routine for you.

Healthy Lifestyle Tip

All adults should set a long-term goal of accumulating physical activity of at least 30 minutes or more of moderate-intensity on most to all days of the week.

Furthermore, aim to improve everyday life habits such as using the stairs instead of the lift, driving farther away, or going to a toilet farther from your office. Reducing sedentary time is a good strategy by undertaking frequent, less strenuous activities to increase activity. You may have the strength to take part in more demanding activities with time.

Pedometers

Self-monitoring instruments are becoming increasingly common and precise. A pedometer is one of the easiest of such self-monitoring devices. Pedometers have all day long quantitative statistics on physical activity. In almost any consumer catalog or retail store, pedometers can be found.

Digi-Walker, Omron, Acumen, Bodytrend, Oregon Science, Sportline, Freestyle, Brookstone, AccuStep, and several more are some of the most common manufactures. Garmin and Timex make speedometer devices that measure steps and speeds using G.P.S. The cost of these clip-on devices ranges from less than $15 to $75.

For everyday exercise, many people get an average of 3,000 steps a day. It is advised to take 10,000 steps a day and work off excess calories for weight-loss. A minimum of 6,000 steps a day is needed to maintain daily safety. Research suggests a 4,000-6,000 step deliberate walk will help with weight-loss. Keeping note of the everyday actions taken in the fitness journal is always a smart idea.

For those more involved in distance commuting, Pedometers may be irritating. Focusing on the number of steps and how to integrate further measures during the day can create a difference for weight reduction as much as it does for physical time. Pedometers allow citizens to consider means of taking further measures over the day.

Because step counting is becoming more popular, advances are being made in the technology behind pedometers. New Pedometers show and reliably count measures. They are meant to be worn on a daily basis, and throughout the day, as a motivation to keep stepping, most are small and wearable.

Pedometers detect your body activity, normally measuring your footsteps with a turned pendulum system, a coiled spring mechanism, and a hairspring mechanism (the least accurate). When you wear it correctly, the unit should be accurate in its count. You might need to experiment on where to wear it. You can measure your step, and then estimate the distance traveled by the pedometer.

Today several pedometers provide multifunctional solutions such as calorie figures, clocks, alarms, stopwatches, pace estimators, readers with seven-day memory or pulse speeds, speech input, and radios.

Accelerometers

While pedometers are quite cost-effective, one of the major shortcomings in the usage of pedometers, however, is that they do not measure movement in strength (how hard) or length (how long) or frequency (how often). Accelerometers are devices capable of objectively measuring physical activity frequency, duration, and intensity.

Accelerometers have high accuracy when measuring physical exercise. There are a number of commercially available accelerometers, or activity monitors, that come from $50 to $1,000 anywhere in a broad range of prices. Some of the inexpensive accelerometers include

BioTrainer and Adidas.

Some of the most complex accelerometers are mainly used in testing or as part of a hospital-based system. Such displays are more versatile in that they display and store more complicated data than pedometers. Some are programmed to transfer the stress rates, gestures, and physical activity habits to a device for study. They may also be used to measure burned calories or spent on oil.

Accelerometers have sophisticated sensors that translate physical activity into an electrical signal relative to the muscle force needed to perform the job. Uniaxial or triaxial measures may be used to find accelerometers. Uniaxial accelerometers assess and may be connected to the trunk or limbs in a single line. Three planes are calculated by triaxial accelerometers: longitudinal, medial-lateral, and anterior-posterior.

Though accelerometers in the precision of physical exercise are a step away from pedometers, they can not detect resistance. Therefore, whether you're practicing in intensity by applying resistance to your cycle by the treadmill, or incorporating an incline to your walking, you won't be able to distinguish the extra endurance amount required to perform the job.

Metabolic Devices

All of the most reliable and costly self-measuring devices are systems that include very advanced calorie burned to measure and reading sensors. Many of these devices have options for subscribing to a Web-based calorie counter system that integrates the amount of burned calories measured by the equipment and your consumed calories that you enter into easy-to-use logs of food.

Such instruments are more precise in calorie measurements, as they use not only accelerometer technology but also heat flux sensors, galvanic skin reaction (to calculate physical exertion and emotional stimuli), and skin temperature gauges. Some also include techniques to monitor heart rate. The integration of both these techniques contributes to a very precise calorie calculation that is expended every day.

Such tools will decide whether you sit in a chair, sleep, exercise, move, raise weights, or run. Many of these instruments are very costly and primarily used for testing, but others are widely used.

Patient-related services often use this equipment. Patients wear the hospital armband and monitor their diet for usually one to two weeks on the Web site or computer-based system. The details will be updated before they report to the facility, and the physicians will be able to communicate with the patients with accurate evidence on metabolic activity trends.

Practitioners may also track patients on automated mobile systems without going face-and-face to provide consultations. Practitioners have the ability to set daily targets for individual patient tailoring programs. They are excellent resources to better track behavior and physical activity critically and to provide the individual with real-time input. One organization that provides this product is SenseWear ®.

4.3 Don't let Lapses become Relapses

Everyone has lapses-but what is the difference between those who can, and who can't, recover? When researchers looked at the National Weight Loss Registry's effective weight losers and contrasted them with those who had lost some of their weight after a year or two, they discovered that only a slight weight increase was hard to reverse: some that had recovered the most weight were least likely to be able to take it off again. That's extra motivation for you to respond on a relapse quickly-and keep checking yourself frequently as well. (If you don't seem to be facing the scale and stop weighing yourself, it's time to do something. First, get on the scale and confront reality. Start measuring weight every day, at the same time. A growing body of evidence supports daily weigh-ins as a way of avoiding weight gain or recovery).

The identification of a "red flag" weight-say, 3 or 5 pounds over the weight limit, is a smart practice. When you see the weight on the scale, find it a warning that a "back on track" approach needs you to respond urgently.

Plan for Relapse Prevention

1. Step back and ask, "What went wrong?" Look from a wider perspective at what brought on the lapse.

3. Remember why you started. Remember of the progress you have made, and how sad you'll be if this one slip-up undoes all your hard work.

2. Calm down. Take a break and a few deep breaths and remind yourself, "One slip-up does not make me a failure."

4. Learn from it. Ponder over what made you return to old habits (your food diary notes can help). What can you do differently next time?

5. Perform your "back on track" strategy right away.

6. Call for backup. You can take help from people who are supportive and who want you to succeed.

4.4 Remember your Why

Know that most people around you are bad and boring when you feel like leaving when they give up on their aspirations!

Know that the fact why few individuals became super-successful relative to the general population is that while they encountered challenges on their path to prosperity, they didn't stop.

Michael Jordan, the iconic basketball player, once claimed, "You have to be able to succeed if you lose." Defeat shouldn't stop you from doing what you set out to achieve.

The Highly Successful don't fear to fail: they will fail many times as long as they get what they want. The desire for their dreams is far greater than the obstacles they face on their path to achieving their goals (discouragements, negative thoughts, and distractions). They opt to stay positive about their goals.

Whenever you're feeling like failing, note that if you give in, your ambitions will never be met.

Remember how people discouraged your dreams!

How they said, you will never make it because you are not good enough!

Will you not want to show you are unique to these people? Do you not want to prove to these people that you have the attitude and mindset of a lion? That you are doing what you set out to do. So the little hurdles will not kill you. So you get what you desire if you want to do everything you like!

Or do you want to make them laugh at you and give negative examples of your failures?

So stop giving it up!

Any of your peers are undermining your aspirations as their achievement tells them they have struggled to fulfill their ambitions. It tells them they settled for mediocre and mediocrity.

David Schwartz says, "This is an environment all around you that is trying to pull you to a second-class street."

Many individuals around you will continue to manipulate you with what's right for you and what you can't accomplish; disregard all these derogatory comments as long as you trust in your path!

Refuse to compare to mediocrity and mediocre. Refuse to create a mental dog condition! Choose to take responsibility for your current state of life and put more effort into your goals because that's the only way you'll get what you've always dreamed of!

Remember what you're doing for when you feel like quitting!

"It doesn't go bad, and you lose your spirit, and you can get angry and give up. They happen to be breaking you down and building you up so you can be all you were meant to be.

Remember the great physics you visualized when you set out to start training at the gym; remember the popular blog you visualized when you set out to become a blogger; the best-selling book you visualized when you decided to become a writer; the billions of dollars you visualized when you started your business.

Don't stop! Don't stop! Recall what you're doing all that for!

If you leave right now, all those wonderful hopes can never be fulfilled! When you give up because of a challenge, you can never enjoy the life of your dreams. Say you're not a quitter, because quitters never win!

The tasks are supposed to keep the mind power. Challenges train you for much tougher future shifts. The hurdles will give you an idea about how to fix your potential problems, so don't have a pessimistic approach to the challenges you encounter. Instead, welcome them positively as they will turn you into the person you've always wanted to be.

Through visualizing the glorious life that awaits them after overcoming their difficulties, the highly productive people typically conquer their problems. The drive for their goals leaves them constantly inspired. They so desperately want results.

Remember that pain is temporary, and gains last forever when you feel like quitting.

"Success is at the end of pain," Eric Thomas.

Never give up on something you really desire. Waiting is challenging yet regrettably more important.

Don't go back down because of the pain you're having. Pain is a part of the process of transforming yourself into the better version you want.

Quitting is for people who don't have heart: people who don't commit to their goals; people who don't want success badly enough to go beyond their limits!

These are the people who are willing to abandon the moment they get tired! They simply do not want to endure the pain of abnormal growth in order to get what they want.

I think you're tired! I know the odds are not your favor! But just remain in the game, for if you leave, nothing wonderful can come.

Know suffering is just fleeting, but achievement is permanent. Give your friend suffering, and you'll get the recognition that you earn!

Seth Godin, a successful entrepreneur, says, "You have to do more than others who have achieved the same goal as yours have done to get what you want."

If even in their worst times, they never leave, so why should you? If they only managed to hold on when it all drops, then why would you abandon your goal? You have not come this far, merely to give up! You did not imagine the vision and set a goal to complete it, only to abandon it halfway!

Don't be a sheep! You're only a lion!

Quitting is defeat! If you quit right now, then you're going to be like most of the world's people living in mediocrity.

You'll be reduced to a weeping hater, and you'll be angry for those who struggled to excel.

Call To Action

Ask yourself the question any time you decide to quit: How badly do you want your goal?

When you're incredibly hungry for your target, then you'll be able to bear all the suffering and overcome all the challenges to fulfill your life of dreams.

If you don't want your vision that badly, so the day the first challenge falls along, you will leave your productive path.

If you want to stay in mediocrity, then quit!

Conclusion

This diet promises to do a quick fix to all of your problems which is very tempting. And there is no doubt that it works wonders and adding Sirt foods in your diet generally is healthy. However, you should keep in mind that diet alone cannot fix all of your problems and maintaining your gains need a consistent discipline in life which is only possible if you don't have a quick fix mindset. You can use this diet plan to quickly see some results and motivate yourself to maintain a better lifestyle which will benefit you in the long term.

Moreover, eating a Sirt food rich diet will boost your immune system and help to prevent future diseases such as obesity. You will feel fresh and active by inclusing foods rich in Sirtuin in your diet. I would suggest that you follow this diet at first but make a habit of adding these foods to your diet and eat healthy in general in future to stick to long term weight management.

If you liked this book and liked the content, I'd like to receive your honest review. Thank you so much.